Primary HIV/AIDS Care

DR CLIVE EVIAN

MBBCH, MFGP, DCH, H.DIP Educ AD, M.MED. (Community Health)

A practical guide
for primary health care personnel
in the clinical and supportive care
of people with HIV/AIDS

Fourth Edition

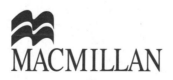

MACMILLAN

Macmillan Education
Between Towns Road, Oxford OX4 3PP
A division of Macmillan Publishers Limited
Companies and representatives throughout the world

www.macmillan-africa.com

ISBN 1-4050-6386-6

Text © Clive Evian 2003, 2005
Design © Jacana Media 2003, 2005

Fourth edition originally published 2003 by
Jacana Media (Pty) Ltd, Johannesburg, South Africa
This edition first published 2005

Typeset by J W Arrowsmith Ltd
Illustrated by Jim Eldridge, Charlotte Peden and Marjorie van Heerden
Cover design by Mark-making Ltd
Cover photograph by Science Photo Library

Although every attempt has been made to ensure that the
management guidelines are safe and correct, the author and
publishers cannot accept any responsibility for errors arising
from the use of this book for any purpose.

Printed and bound in Malaysia

2009 2008 2007 2006 2005
10 9 8 7 6 5 4 3 2 1

DEDICATION

I dedicate this book to a late friend, mentor and editor – Janet Orlek – who gave me so much insight into the reading difficulties experienced by those whose second language is English, and who taught me how to write in simple, plain English. My original experience working with her as my editor for the Primary Clinical Care series enabled me to write this book.
I miss her skills and her laughter.

*"AIDS makes me feel alive. Every day I am thankful and grateful for being alive. I breathe and enjoy the fresh air; I notice the blue skies and the colourful flowers; I feel the warmth of the sun; I am **living** with AIDS."*
(A person with advanced HIV/AIDS 1990)

"It is not the HIV virus which is killing me or making my life not worth living, but the bad attitudes of people towards me and their rejection of me."
(A person with HIV infection, December 1992)

"I am a young man and I need and want a close and intimate relationship with a woman, yet whenever I tell her that we must use a condom, because I have HIV, she is no longer interested in a sexual relationship. It is very difficult living with HIV."
(A man with early HIV infection)

"Now that I have HIV, it makes me feel that I am living outside of the world. Every day and every hour and every minute I am aware that I am infected with HIV."
(A well patient trying to cope with HIV/AIDS 1998)

*"**Struggle:**
To make a vigorous effort, in unfavourable circumstances, to overcome difficulties and problems."*

CONTENTS

FOREWORD

Having well-trained, knowledgeable and highly motivated health professionals working in service delivery at all levels is crucial for effective management of the health aspects of the HIV epidemic. Families living with HIV and AIDS desperately need access to reliable, accessible and affordable treatment and care. These resources will help them cope with the impact of this disease on their lives and their children's future. Tragically, in many parts of Africa, health services have been devastated by under-funding, poor morale, and loss of staff through illness, death and migration, often as a consequence of the HIV epidemic itself.

Health professionals need many inputs to provide good services for people living with HIV and AIDS. They need leadership, supervision, training, resources, drugs, incentives, motivation, and community support. The continuum-of-care approach builds from hospital or health centre to community home-based care, with management of sexually transmitted infections, family planning and reproductive healthcare, tuberculosis services and outreach, voluntary counselling and testing services, prevention of HIV transmission to infants and linkages to support groups. Clients and patients, as well as carers and health workers, need information at every point on how to put these services to best use.

This book is an excellent practical guide for health professionals in addressing HIV from the primary care perspective, equipping readers with the knowledge they need to provide HIV services in the integrated fashion described above. It also works well as a training guide for managers and supervisors of primary care professionals. The style of language and layout is accessible and user-friendly not only for health professionals at various stages of knowledge, but also offering a structure for providing basic information for patients and client groups.

It provides chapters on testing and counselling for HIV, management of HIV in women and children, as well as prevention of HIV transmission to infants, the linkages between other sexually transmitted infections and HIV, and tuberculosis and HIV. Especially useful are sections on managing pain relief for people with AIDS, as well as occupational concerns for health workers and HIV transmission.

The publication of this Macmillan edition is particularly timely because of increasing interest in provision of anti-retroviral therapy (ART) in Africa. Availability of ART was limited in the past to the private sector in many countries, but has become much more centre stage through the public sector as international campaigns have brought the cost of treatment down. Several countries have started developing ART programmes. The recent launch of the World Health Organisation's $5.5 billion plan aims to provide treatment for three million HIV-positive people by 2005. It also calls for the training of 100,000 health care workers, and the refocusing of 10,000 clinics in developing countries to treat HIV- and AIDS-related illness, using some common anti-retroviral drug combinations. In this edition Clive Evian has included up-to-date information on treating opportunistic infections and the use of ART, but as one part of an integrated service that includes prevention, counselling, testing and management of other HIV-related conditions including palliative care. This edition therefore provides a vital resource for this campaign.

I am confident that health workers, and indeed all involved in the support and care of families living with HIV and AIDS, will find this book useful. It makes an important contribution to the urgent action needed in addressing HIV throughout the African continent.

Dr Sunanda Ray MB BS, MSc, MPH, MFPHM (UK)
Consultant in Public Health and Communicable Disease Control, formerly Director of SAfAIDS, the Southern Africa HIV/AIDS information service
June 2004

ACKNOWLEDGEMENTS

Many people have contributed in various ways to help develop and produce the original version and the later editions of this book. I wish to thank all those who have contributed in one way or another.

I am mostly indebted to Jenny Prangley for her dedication and skills at editing the book. It is indeed a privilege to have worked with Jenny, and her insight, patience and commitment have gone a long way to making this book readable, and especially accessible, to those whose first language is not English. I would also like to acknowledge the rest of the Jacana team, especially Julia Gault, Mike Martin, Angela McClelland and Brett Rogers for work on this edition.

I am grateful to the Southern African Journal of HIV Medicine, the official journal of the Southern African HIV Clinicians Society, which provided much of the updated material for this edition. This journal is highly recommended to all practitioners involved in HIV care.

My acknowledgements and thanks to the doctors, nurses, health care workers and others who assisted in the development of this book since its inception:
Ron Ballard, Daynia Ballot, Pierre Brouard, Mark Cotton, Mary Crewe, Cindy Firnhaber, Harry Hausler, Shirley Henen, Stan Henen, Justus Hofmeyer, Greg Hussey, Ute Jentsch, Makie Kunene, Gary Maartens, Des Martin, James McIntyre, Neil McKerow, Steve Miller, Stephanie Moore, Noreen Napper, Graham Neilsen, Charlotte Peden, Inez Pinto, Claire Pooley, Ian Sanne, Sawera Singh, Ray Smego, Alan Smith, Bruce Sparks, David Spencer, Malcolm Steinberg, Anne Strätling and Marjorie van Heerden.

Finally, thanks to my wife Sara for her unique personal support, and to my children Nikia, Shira, Tahl and Shai, and my mom Sonia for their patience while I diverted many hours of family time to attend to the book.

"We have failed to translate our scientific progress into action where it is most needed – in communities in the developing world regions, the poorest regions of the globe. This is a global injustice which cannot be tolerated. It is a travesty of human rights on a global scale. The world must do more, much more, on every front in the fight against AIDS. This means dramatically expanding on prevention efforts, but the most striking inequality is our failure to provide life-saving treatment to millions of people who need it most. It is our view that the single most important step we must now take is to provide access to treatment throughout the developing world – there is no excuse for delay."

Nelson Mandela, 2nd International Conference on Care and Pathogenesis, Paris, July 2003

INTRODUCTION

Primary HIV/AIDS Care was first published in 1993 when HIV was still a relatively new disease raising many challenges. It is a disease which usually targets the most physically active and those on whom others depend; a disease that raises many difficulties, uncertainties and fears; and a disease that triggers a cascade of personal losses culminating in the most precious of all possessions – one's life.

We had much to learn about the virus, the disease and how people and society would respond to the epidemic. There were only three anti-retroviral drugs available, they were too expensive for most people, and there were too few combinations for effective long-term therapy. Yet despite the limitations and difficulties, we moved forward, we did our best and we kept hope alive.

There have been so many new discoveries and strategies for managing people with HIV/AIDS. We can now offer people with HIV much better care and hope for longer and healthier lives. There are many more new anti-retroviral medicines, which are much cheaper and are becoming more accessible to African countries. HIV has now become a manageable chronic disease. Health care workers and the services are becoming more familiar and experienced in diagnosing and treating HIV and its related conditions. We can honestly offer people with HIV real hope, and towards this end, it is very exciting to be able to provide this updated and revised edition of this book. We are confident that it will contribute to the improved care and outlook for people with HIV/AIDS.

This manual has attempted to provide primary health care personnel with a user-friendly guide and approach to the medical care of people with HIV/AIDS. Besides the purely medical assessment and care, it also addresses such issues as HIV testing, counselling, specific needs of women and children and health care workers, as well as management of pain and of those who are terminally ill. Current approaches and recommendations for the use of anti-retroviral therapy are highlighted in all relevant sections. The book also deals with the prevention of peri-natally acquired HIV and post-exposure prophylaxis (prevention). As tuberculosis and other sexually transmitted infections are so closely associated with HIV, these conditions have also been included.

While writing the book I have also been acutely aware of the realities and diversity of African countries. Health care workers and their patients are located in a wide spectrum of economic and social contexts. These range from highly developed urban societies to isolated rural and traditional communities; from well-resourced and advanced technological facilities to those in poorer and low-resourced areas; from highly educated and informed individuals to those who are illiterate and with minimal or no education or access to information about HIV. Primary care personnel also differ in their training, qualifications and experience. This may range from university trained, specialised, primary care doctors to primary care nurses and assistants with much less training, back-up and support. The need is therefore to provide a range of care options from simple, affordable and available therapies to the new, more sophisticated (and costly) options. We have also tried to make the text more accessible to those for whom English is a second language.

Besides doctors and nurse clinicians, the book will be valuable to other primary care practitioners such as counsellors, social workers, home care, traditional and alternative health care providers, educators, and other therapists. Patients themselves may find the information helps them to understand the various clinical issues and peculiarities relating to their disease.

We are continually learning about this disease, and some opinions and therapies may differ from those provided in this book, or there may be alternative approaches. We have tried to give the essential and most widely accepted approaches and therapies. Readers are urged to keep abreast with new developments and with local therapies and approaches to HIV care, and where necessary to adapt the recommendations provided in this book.

Primary HIV/AIDS Care is a practical guide and a departure point especially for those who are unfamiliar or relatively new to medically managing or caring for people with HIV/AIDS and for those in training. It will also serve as a useful reference point in the clinical setting.

The images and descriptions of AIDS are too often morbid and extremely bleak, and while we should never underestimate the seriousness and potential devastation of this disease, we must also not forget the human side. This aspect of HIV/AIDS has brought out the very best in people, and there are many courageous stories about people affected by the disease, and the relationships that have been deepened and enriched through caring, understanding and compassion. The enthusiasm of many people throughout the world in their efforts to overcome this disease and the epidemic is enlightening and exciting.

> **The epidemic has highlighted the fact that our world needs to change. More generosity, compassion, care, loyalty and respect for each other are needed. I hope this book will help, even in a very small way, to contribute to this change.**

Readers are welcome to share experiences, ideas and knowledge through correspondence with the author (e-mail address below).

Clive Evian
drclive@icon.co.za

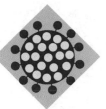

Chapter 1

AIDS, A NEW AND UNIQUE CHALLENGE

The history of AIDS

AIDS and primary health care

The I IIV virus

How HIV causes immune-deficiency

The production of HIV antibodies
in response to HIV infection

The development of signs and symptoms
of HIV infection

The history of AIDS

The acquired immune-deficiency syndrome (AIDS) is a relatively new and unique disease. It was first described in America, in 1981, after a number of men had developed a rare pneumonia caused by a parasite called *Pneumocystis carinii*.

These men were all previously healthy, between 20 and 45 years of age and homosexually-orientated.

They had all developed severe immune-deficiency which led to the development of this rare pneumonia.

Soon afterwards, in central Africa, health care workers were discovering a new disease, causing severe weight loss and diarrhoea, which they called 'Slims disease'. This was also due to immune-deficiency and it was present in heterosexually-orientated people. More and more people began developing this illness and other conditions associated with immune-deficiency.

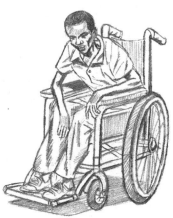

Advanced AIDS

- ◆ In September 1983, scientists discovered the human immune-deficiency virus (HIV) to be the cause of this new disease, called AIDS.

- ◆ In 1985, the ELISA HIV antibody test became available.

- ◆ In 1987, the first anti-retroviral drug (ARV) AZT was approved for use.

- ◆ In 1994, ARVs were used to prevent mother to child HIV transmission (MTCT).

- ◆ In 1995, triple-drug anti-retroviral therapy (ART), Highly Active ARV therapy (HAART), was introduced.

- ◆ In 1998/9, HIV vaccine trials were begun.

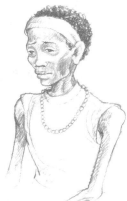

Slims disease

Now, more than 20 years after HIV was first described, millions of people have become infected worldwide, and AIDS has become the world's most serious public health problem. Africa has one of the most severe HIV/AIDS epidemics in the world.

AIDS and primary health care

HIV is now a manageable chronic disease

Managing people with HIV/AIDS now includes:

◆ HIV viral suppression with ART medication

◆ Delaying the onset of serious immune deficiency, opportunistic infections and AIDS

◆ Managing and supporting patients to adhere strictly to their ART drug regimen

◆ Avoiding and managing drug side effects and toxicity

◆ Avoiding and managing emerging ARV drug resistance

◆ Preventing mother to child HIV transmission (MTCT) with ART

◆ Counselling affected people

◆ Supporting and caring for people who are ill and dying

◆ Using prevention strategies to control the spread of HIV

Most of the problems associated with HIV infection can be dealt with at the primary care level. The management and care of people with AIDS will need to be incorporated into the overall primary health care service. These services must be accessible and affordable to those who need them.

Every opportunity must be taken to educate people in the prevention of the disease, and in the support and acceptance of those who are infected with HIV.

Part of the overall strategy to control the spread of HIV must include the treatment and care of people with sexually transmitted infections (STIs), and the reduction of risky sexual activity.

Tuberculosis is one of the most common HIV-associated serious life-threatening diseases. Care of people with active TB will become an increasing need.

> **Having a sexually transmitted infection assists in the transmission of the HIV virus into the body.**

HIV can also be passed from a mother to her unborn child during pregnancy, childbirth and breast feeding (*see Chapter 10*). Many of these infections can also be prevented through specific interventions and obstetric and infant feeding practices. This will place extra demands on antenatal, childbirth, family planning and child-care services.

Finally, there will be a need to develop support services to manage people at home as well as in the hospitals and clinics.

> **The care and support of people with HIV/AIDS must be incorporated into the overall primary health care services. The improvement and accessibility of care for patients with sexually transmitted infections is also an urgent priority.**

The HIV virus

HIV (human immuno-deficiency virus) was discovered to be the cause of AIDS in 1983. It is unclear from where the virus came, or why it appeared. There is evidence that the virus has been around for at least 20 years, and it is possible that it was present even before this time.

It has recently been discovered that the HIV virus developed from a mutation of the simian virus which infected chimpanzees. The virus later jumped to monkeys, and from monkeys to humans.

The movement and migration of people across large distances, socio-economic instability, intravenous drug use and multiple partner sexual activity has enabled the virus to spread rapidly worldwide.

HIV is a retrovirus

A retrovirus can undergo an unusual biological process in which the genetic material, in the form of single-stranded RNA, can be converted to double-stranded DNA. In nature DNA usually makes RNA. An enzyme called **reverse transcriptase** enables the virus to perform this reverse action. A number of ART drugs are targeted at this enzyme, such as zidovudine, didanosine and stavudine etc.

More recently a new group of drugs has become available to target the protease reaction in the replication process of the virus. These 'protease inhibitors', such as indinavir, ritonavir etc. have added a new dimension to anti-retroviral therapy (ART) (*see Chapter 5*).

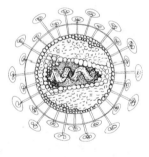

HIV virus

The virus has a circular shape. Its core RNA genetic material is covered by an envelope that has many, small, glycoprotein projections on its surface. These projections have an attraction to certain target cells, with so-called CD4 receptor sites.

These CD4 receptors are present on various types of blood cells including:

◆ Lymphocytes, such as CD4 (helper) T lymphocytes

◆ Macrophages

◆ Monocytes

◆ Tissue cells (such as dendritic cells present in the genital tract and ano-rectal region)

◆ Certain brain cells (glial cells)

◆ Some other cells as well

After binding to the CD4 receptor, the viral genetic material enters the host's cell (e.g. a CD4 cell). With the reverse transcriptase reaction, as described above, the virus's DNA copy becomes incorporated into the host cell. Later, when new virus particles are made, they bud off from the host cell, enter the blood stream and infect more cells. In this process, the host cells (such as the CD4 T lymphocytes) are damaged and destroyed.

Life cycle of HIV and site of action of ARVs

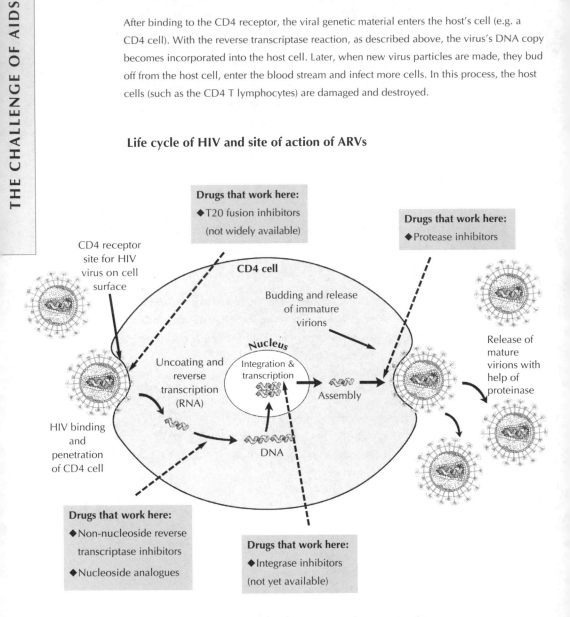

Drugs that work here:
◆ T20 fusion inhibitors
(not widely available)

Drugs that work here:
◆ Protease inhibitors

CD4 receptor site for HIV virus on cell surface

CD4 cell

Budding and release of immature virions

Nucleus

Uncoating and reverse transcription (RNA)

Integration & transcription

Assembly

Release of mature virions with help of proteinase

HIV binding and penetration of CD4 cell

DNA

Drugs that work here:
◆ Non-nucleoside reverse transcriptase inhibitors
◆ Nucleoside analogues

Drugs that work here:
◆ Integrase inhibitors
(not yet available)

Note: The size of the virus has been artificially enlarged in this illustration. Relative to the size of the cell, it would be approximately the size of this full stop.

How HIV causes immune-deficiency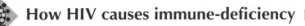

◆ The HIV virus attacks and slowly destroys the immune system

HIV enters and destroys important cells which control and support the immune system.

After entering the body, HIV attaches to the CD4 receptors, mainly on dendritic cells and T lymphocytes, known as 'helper' cells (or T4 or CD4 cells). HIV can also attach to other cells, such as monocytes, macrophages and others, if they possess a CD4 receptor on their surface.

After attachment and entry into the CD4 cells, the HIV finally destroys the cell or results in dysfunction of the cell.

The CD4 (T4) helper cells are very important in the regulation and control of the immune response

- ◆ Directly, or indirectly, they protect the body from invasion by certain bacteria, viruses, fungi and parasites.
- ◆ They clear away a number of cancer cells.
- ◆ They are also involved in the production of substances involved in the body's defence (such as interleukins and interferon).
- ◆ They also influence the development and function of monocytes and macrophages, which act as scavenger cells in the immune system.

This all means that some of the most important cells of the body's immune or defence system are destroyed. The immune system is very well established and is very powerful. It takes the HIV virus a number of years to destroy enough of the immune system to cause immune-deficiency and immune-incompetence.

> **After a long period of infection, usually 3 – 7 years, large numbers of virus particles are produced, which destroy enough of the immune cells and lead to immune-deficiency. When a person is immune-deficient, the body has difficulty defending itself against many infections and some cancers.**

It is possible to monitor the development and degree of immune-deficiency by doing laboratory tests. *This is discussed in more detail in Chapter 5.*

◆ Response to HIV infection

There is a wide variation in how people respond and react to HIV. In some the virus may cause immune damage and illness earlier than others. It appears that in a small proportion of infected people (about 5%), there may be no development of immune-deficiency at all.

There are two general types of responses:

Rapid progressors

◆ People who are rapid progressors usually develop immune-deficiency within 5 – 7 years after infection
   – for some this may be shortened to 3 – 4 years.

◆ People who have a rapidly progressing illness have a very active and 'aggressive' viral strain. Their bodies cannot suppress the virus sufficiently to delay or stop the progress of the disease.

Slow progressors

◆ Slow progressors generally remain well and active without any disease, and with very little or absent immune-deficiency.

◆ They may remain well for 10 – 15 years or more.

In a very small proportion (about 5%) of HIV-infected people, there is no obvious disease progression. For some reason (usually genetic) these individuals do not develop immune-deficiency despite being infected with HIV.

There are complex reasons why some people are rapid and others slow progressors. It is related to:

   – different HIV viral strains
   – the dosage of infection
   – the body's response to the virus
   – the general health status of the individual

For this reason it is important to prevent repeated infections, and to try to reduce the initial viral load (*see Chapter 5*).

◆ When does someone have AIDS?

A person is described as having AIDS when the HIV-related immune-deficiency is so severe that various life-threatening, opportunistic infections and/or cancers occur. These conditions only occur because the immune system is weakened.

These infections and cancers are called 'opportunistic diseases', because they take the opportunity provided by the lowered immune state i.e. if the immunity is normal, these diseases would not usually occur. *This is discussed in more detail in Chapter 6.*

The scientific case definition of AIDS and the staging of the disease can be found on pages 118 – 120.

The production of HIV antibodies in response to HIV infection

In response to the HIV infection:

- The immune system develops antibodies to HIV.
- These antibodies are not able to overcome or destroy the virus.
- They can usually be detected in the blood stream 4 – 6 weeks after infection.

These antibodies form the basis for the HIV antibody blood test (*see Chapter 4*).
The HIV antibody test is often the only way to know if a person is definitely infected with the HIV virus. This is especially true in the early or asymptomatic period.

The development of signs and symptoms of HIV infection

It may take 3 – 7 years, or even more, for a person who is HIV-infected to develop immune-deficiency and HIV-related medical conditions. This means that most people can be infected with HIV yet remain well for a long period of time. During this time, a positive HIV test is usually the only way of knowing that the person is infected with HIV.

Despite a person being well during this time, he/she is able to spread the virus. Later, when the immune system is weak and unable to adequately defend the body, signs and symptoms develop.

These signs and symptoms are usually due to:

- New infections, especially opportunistic infections
- Reactivation of old, inactive or dormant infections, such as tuberculosis, herpes or unusual cancers
- The HIV virus itself and its impact on various organs and tissues in the body

The disease may progress more rapidly in individuals who are already chronically ill or who have a poor health status such as:

- chronic disease
- recurrent infections
- anaemia
- malnutrition and nutritional deficiency
- repeated pregnancies without adequate recovery between each pregnancy
- malaria
- TB

The nature of the epidemic, how the HIV virus is spread, and some of the social and economic determinants (factors) of the epidemic are briefly discussed in the following chapter.

Additional notes for new developments

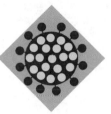

Chapter 2

THE SPREAD OF
HIV INFECTION

How HIV is spread

The most infectious phases for HIV-infected people

Casual contact does not appear to spread HIV

The AIDS epidemic

The influence of poverty and low socio-economic
conditions on the spread of HIV

◆ How HIV is spread

HIV is generally spread in three ways:

◆ Via sexual intercourse

◆ When HIV-infected blood is passed directly into the body

◆ From mother to child during pregnancy, childbirth
and via breast feeding

These are discussed in more detail below.

◆ HIV is transmitted through sexual intercourse

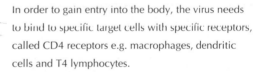

HIV is transmitted from one person to another through the most intimate of
contact – sexual intercourse. The virus is found in high quantities
in the sexual fluids (semen and vaginal fluid) of people with
HIV infection.

In order to gain entry into the body, the virus needs
to bind to specific target cells with specific receptors,
called CD4 receptors e.g. macrophages, dendritic
cells and T4 lymphocytes.

These receptors enable the virus to successfully attach and gain entry into the
body's cells. The receptor cells are plentiful in the lining of the genital tract and the
ano-rectal area.

Although the virus can be found in other body fluids, such as saliva, urine and sweat,
the quantities of HIV in these fluids are usually too low for successful transmission.
HIV infection has not been reported to have been acquired via a healthy mouth or
respiratory tract. However it may be possible to transmit the virus if there are fresh
sores or inflammation in the mouth. The skin does not have CD4 receptor cells on
the surface, and HIV cannot enter through normal, intact (undamaged) skin.

HIV is not spread via non sexual, casual contact between people. Individuals who
have not had sexual intercourse, or received or shared blood (or blood products)
could not have acquired HIV infection. Children remain free of HIV infection even
after intimate contact (hugging, kissing) with their infected parents, and after sharing
common utensils, baths, linen etc.

The presence of other sexually transmitted infections makes the sexual transmission of HIV easier

Other genital ulcers or sores, caused by syphilis, chancroid, gonorrhoea, herpes virus and other sexually transmitted infections (STIs) are thought to assist the HIV virus in entering the body.

◆ It appears that the virus can enter through the ulcer itself, and attach to the CD4 receptors. These are present on various inflammatory cells, in and around the ulcer.

◆ HIV can also spread, from the exposed surface of the ulcer, to the genital tract of the sexual partner.

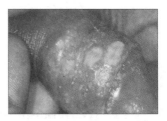

Genital ulcer

◆ Other STIs, such as gonorrhoea and chlamidial infection, also cause an inflammatory response in the genital tract with a migration of inflammatory cells to the infection. This also promotes the successful transmission of HIV (*see also Chapter 12 on STIs and HIV*).

◆ The discharges that occur with many STIs have a very high concentration of HIV if the person with the STI is HIV positive.

> **The effective treatment of genital ulcer disease (syphilis, chancroid, herpes) and other STIs can play an important role in the control and prevention of HIV infection.**

Anal or vaginal intercourse

Anal sex appears to be the sexual practice carrying the highest risk for transmitting the HIV virus. The lining of the anal-rectal area is relatively easily torn during anal intercourse. This allows the virus to enter the body more easily. Vaginal sex is also an effective form of transmission. Vaginal and anal sex is safer if a condom is correctly used.

It is not yet certain whether anyone has developed HIV infection through oral sex alone, however it may have some risk. Non-penetrative sex, such as sex between the thighs and masturbation, are considered safer.

◆ HIV and blood transmission

Infection can also occur if HIV-infected blood gains entry into the body. For infection to occur, the blood from an HIV-infected person must bypass the barrier of the skin and enter directly into the body.

This means that HIV-infected blood becomes a high risk when passed into the body in the following ways:

◆ Through a blood transfusion

◆ Via blood-contaminated needles, syringes, razor blades and other sharp instruments

◆ Through intravenous drug use (sharing of needles and syringes)

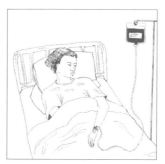

Blood transfusions

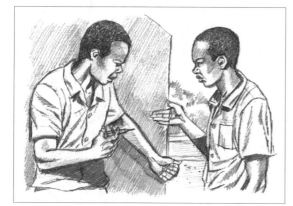

Sharing needles during intravenous drug use

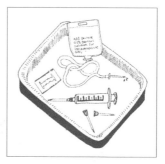

Contaminated needles and instruments

◆ It is also possible, but very rare, for HIV to enter the body through an open skin wound or sore.

It is important for all blood to be tested for HIV before it is regarded as safe for blood transfusion. It is also important for health care workers to be careful when using sharp instruments, taking blood, putting up drips, doing invasive surgical procedures and handling blood-stained dressings, linen or instruments.

The necessary safety precautions that health care workers need to take to prevent infection, and the management of occupationally acquired HIV exposure (needlestick injuries etc.) is discussed in Chapter 15.

THE SPREAD OF HIV

◆ Mother to child HIV transmission (MTCT)

In recent years a better understanding of MTCT and the ways to prevent it have developed.

Pregnancy and childbirth

A pregnant mother, who is infected with HIV, can pass on the virus to her infant during pregnancy and childbirth. Research has shown that there is a 20% – 40% chance that the infant will become HIV-infected. This means, that if a mother is HIV positive, there is approximately a 1 in 3 chance that her infant will be born with HIV infection.

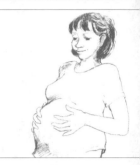

Pregnancy

It is not yet clear why some women pass the virus on to their babies and why others do not.

It appears that a woman is more likely to transmit the virus to her foetus during pregnancy if:

◆ She becomes infected just before or during the pregnancy

◆ She has a high HIV viral load

◆ She has symptomatic HIV disease

◆ She has a low CD4 count

Childbirth

See Chapter 10.

This means that a symptomatic mother is more likely to pass on the virus than a mother who has no symptoms of HIV disease.

There are many ways to reduce the risk of MTCT during labour. These include:
 – the use of ART during pregnancy and labour, and giving the newborn baby ART during the first 6 weeks after birth
 – avoiding unnecessary rupture of membranes and episiotomy
 – avoiding prolonged labour
 – minimising trauma to the foetus
 – the mode of delivery (Caesarean section)

These and other methods are discussed in more detail in Chapter 10.

THE SPREAD OF HIV

Breast feeding

The issue of infant feeding in low resourced and low socio-economic communities is a complex issue. There is a definite HIV transmission risk to the foetus from breast feeding, and there is also a potential risk to the foetus from gastro-enteritis, malnutrition and other infective conditions from unsafe formula feeding.

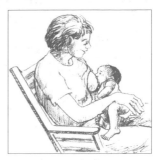

Breast feeding

Health care workers will need to carefully inform and advise mothers. Balancing these risks and choosing the most appropriate feeding method is a new challenge to health care workers and to the mothers.

MTCT and its prevention is discussed more fully in Chapter 10.

 ## The most infectious phases for HIV-infected people

A person is most likely to *pass on* the HIV virus during the following phases:

◆ Soon after becoming infected with the HIV virus (in the first 4 – 8 weeks)

◆ When there is a high HIV viral load

◆ During the later phase of the infection, when symptoms of HIV infection/AIDS appear

This is because there are larger quantities of virus in the blood stream at these times. Remember that it is possible to transmit HIV **anytime** during the disease.

> **HIV-infected people are considered most infectious soon after acquiring the HIV infection and during the AIDS (symptomatic) phase.**

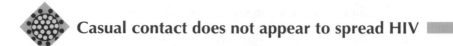

Casual contact does not appear to spread HIV

There is no good evidence that HIV is spread through normal, everyday, casual contact between individuals.

- The HIV virus is not stable and does not survive for long periods outside the human body.

- The virus cannot penetrate normal intact skin and does not readily enter through a healthy mouth or eye.

- Also the virus is not present in high enough quantities in the saliva and urine to cause infection.

- A person with a healthy genital tract is less likely to acquire HIV than a person with genital disease (such as an STI).

HIV is not normally transmitted by the following means:

- Airborne routes, such as coughing, sneezing, laughing, talking and kissing

- Simple skin contact, such as hand-shaking, hugging and touching etc.

- Food, water, or on plates, cups, spoons, toilets, baths, pools and showers etc.

- Towels, bed linen, clothes, etc.

- Insects, such as mosquitoes, are not known to spread HIV from one person to another.

HIV is NOT spread by casual, everyday, non-sexual contact.

THE SPREAD OF HIV

HIV is NOT spread by casual, everyday, non-sexual contact.

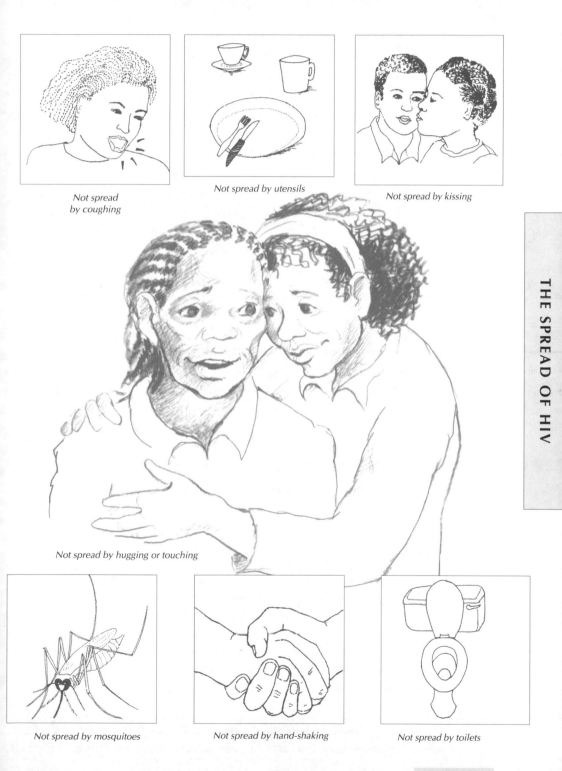

Not spread
by coughing

Not spread by utensils

Not spread by kissing

Not spread by hugging or touching

Not spread by mosquitoes

Not spread by hand-shaking

Not spread by toilets

The AIDS epidemic

◆ HIV is most commonly spread via sexual intercourse (90%). As a result of this, HIV/AIDS is most common in people between 15 and 50 years old.

◆ Men and women are both affected. Women seem more vulnerable to infection than men, and young girls are known to become infected earlier than boys. This is because girls often become sexually active earlier than boys, and older men tend to have sex with young girls. This is especially true in countries with lots of men migrating to the cities for employment.

◆ In America and Europe, most of those first infected were homosexual men and intravenous drug users. But now, in these areas, the infection has also spread to heterosexual people.

◆ The spread of AIDS via infected blood is less common. The sharing of needles and syringes by intravenous drug users causes approximately 30% of HIV infections in countries where intravenous drug-use is common (e.g. the USA and Europe).

◆ Health services can also spread HIV infection if the blood transfusions are not first tested and screened for HIV, or if blood-contaminated needles and equipment are used. This form of spread is more common in poorer countries. In countries where all the blood donated for transfusion is tested, there are very few infections as a result of blood transfusion.

◆ AIDS is also found in children between the age of birth and approximately 10 years, and sometimes even older. This is mainly due to the transmission of infection during pregnancy and childbirth.

AIDS is a world-wide disease

By the end of 2003, it was estimated that there were about 40 million people worldwide who were infected with the HIV virus. Three million people died of AIDS in that same year.

AIDS in sub-Saharan Africa

Roughly 70% of the world's HIV infection is found in sub-Saharan Africa. It is estimated that up to 29 million adults and children are living with HIV, and that a further 3 – 4 million are infected each year. Approximately 2.3 million people in sub-Saharan Africa died of AIDS in 2003. It is estimated that only 50 000 people in Africa had access to anti-retroviral drugs in 2002, but some African countries are making determined efforts to improve this access. Recent years have also seen greater political commitment and increased funding aimed at reversing the epidemic.

HIV has spread to all parts of the world and is the most serious public health problem.

The influence of poverty and low socio-economic conditions on the spread of HIV

AIDS and other sexually transmitted infections are often more common in lower socio-economic countries.

Some of the reasons why low socio-economic conditions promote the spread of sexually transmitted infections are as follows:

◆ **The relationships between men and women suffer**. Women are often exploited and have a more inferior status than men. In many communities **women have very little control over their sexual lives, and the ways to prevent STIs**. Poverty often makes this sexual exploitation worse, and this further contributes to the spread of sexually transmitted infections.

◆ **High unemployment promotes migrant work and family disruption**. People leave their homes and therefore their loved ones, friends, familiar surroundings and local community life. In the far-away places, migrants often find themselves in lonely, unfavourable, hostile or alienating environments. There is a natural need for sex and intimacy resulting in multiple-partner sexual relationships.

◆ **Women are often forced to sell sex** to earn precious money for food and basic needs, and to help raise their children. Young girls may sell sex to older men.

◆ People in poor living conditions **often do not have easy access to health care services**. Sexually transmitted infections often go untreated and spread more easily.

◆ **Poor education and low literacy levels** help to keep people ignorant of the ways and means to avoid diseases like AIDS.

◆ People often drink too much **alcohol**, or smoke **dagga** (marijuana, zoll, ganja), or use drugs to escape from the everyday hardships. This also encourages people to become 'loose', and to have sex with different people.

◆ **Crime and violence** is also common in cities and towns, and these further **stress family and community life.**

◆ Many of the problems described above also result in the **breakdown of the usual traditions, customs, beliefs and cultural practices in a community**. These practices usually determine the accepted sexual behaviour and constraints in a society. When these are broken down, it often results in multiple sexual partners and indiscriminate sexual behaviour.

See diagram on the following page.

> **There are many reasons why HIV is spreading.**
> **Prevention and care measures need to take account of the socio-economic factors that promote the spread of HIV.**

The natural expected clinical course, from the onset of HIV infection, to the development of AIDS, is discussed in the next chapter.

THE SPREAD OF HIV

Poverty creates the conditions and environment which contribute to the spread of HIV

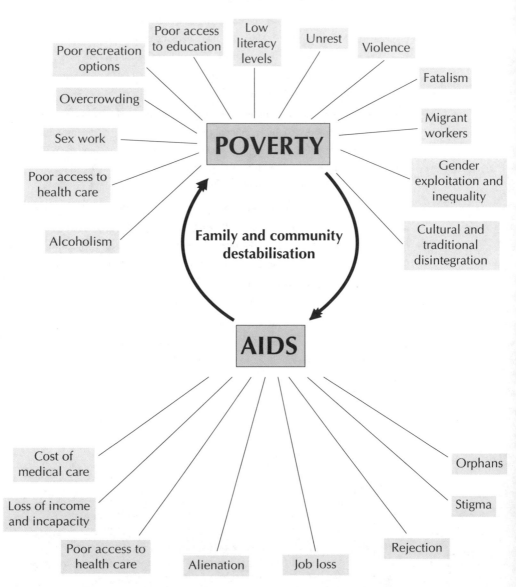

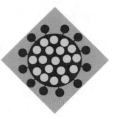

Chapter 3

FROM HIV INFECTION
TO AIDS

An introduction to the development of immune-deficiency and
the progression to AIDS

Early (Primary) HIV infection

Clinical latent or 'silent' infection – the asymptomatic phase

Minor HIV-related symptoms – the minor symptomatic phase

HIV-related disease – the symptomatic phase

Severe HIV-related disease – AIDS, the severe symptomatic phase

An introduction to the development of immune-deficiency and the progression to AIDS

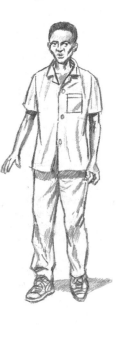

A person who becomes infected with HIV will usually go through various clinical stages that occur over a long period of time (usually 5 – 12 years).

These stages occur with the patient:

◆ Being well with no symptoms of disease (asymptomatic)

◆ To having mild disease episodes

◆ To having severe illness (symptomatic)

◆ And finally with the patient dying

HIV slowly damages the immune system, and the appearance and manifestation of disease is usually related to the degree of immune-deficiency and the HIV viral load in the body.

Anti-retroviral therapy (ART) can significantly change the course of the disease, and prolong the well and asymptomatic phase.

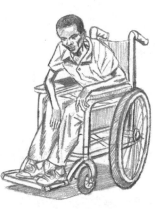

The World Health Organisation Staging System and the Center for Disease Control case definition of HIV/AIDS are outlined on pages 118 – 120.

Severe symptomatic disease is almost always related to advanced immune-deficiency.

FROM HIV TO AIDS

The state of the immune system is the best predictor of the patient's risk of developing symptomatic disease. Measuring the CD4 (helper T cells) is currently regarded as the best indicator of immune-deficiency in HIV disease, and is used to monitor the immune status of the person.

In the absence of a CD4 cell count, the lymphocyte count can also be helpful but it is less specific and less accurate. Even in the absence of these tests, the health care worker may rely on the presence of HIV-related signs and symptoms, such as thrush, shingles, Kaposi's sarcoma etc., as indicators of advanced immune-deficiency.

The table and graph below outline the development of the various phases of HIV infection in relation to the immune status (the CD4 count/lymphocyte count).

AIDS is the advanced, late and final stage of HIV infection, and is associated with severe immune-deficiency.

THE RELATIONSHIP BETWEEN THE IMMUNE STATUS, THE CD4 COUNT, THE LYMPHOCYTE COUNT & THE PRESENCE OF SYMPTOMATIC DISEASE		
Clinical condition	**CD4 cell count**	**Lymphocyte count**
Well with no symptoms	more than 500 – 600 cells/mm³	more than 2 500 cells/mm³
Minor symptoms	350 – 500 cells/mm³	1 250 – 2 500 cells/mm³
Major symptoms and some opportunistic diseases	200 – 350 cells/mm³	500 – 1 250 cells/mm³
AIDS	less than 200 cells/mm³	500 – 1 250 cells/mm³

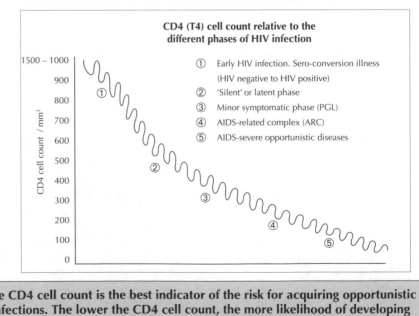

CD4 (T4) cell count relative to the different phases of HIV infection

① Early HIV infection. Sero-conversion illness (HIV negative to HIV positive)
② 'Silent' or latent phase
③ Minor symptomatic phase (PGL)
④ AIDS-related complex (ARC)
⑤ AIDS-severe opportunistic diseases

The CD4 cell count is the best indicator of the risk for acquiring opportunistic infections. The lower the CD4 cell count, the more likelihood of developing opportunistic infections and other HIV-related diseases.

◆ HIV viral load

The HIV viral load refers to the level of HIV virus in the blood stream. This is a relatively new test which has more recently become available (in some places). The HIV viral load is tested by the HIV RNA PCR quantification test.

This test and its interpretation is discussed in more detail in Chapters 4 and 5.

The viral load usually rises to high levels soon after HIV infection (within the first week). This is due to a very rapid multiplication and replication of the virus after infection. As the body develops antibodies to HIV, the virus level in the blood decreases, as the virus is mainly swept into the lymph nodes. The decline in the HIV load usually coincides with the time of sero-conversion and the primary HIV infection described below.

Viral load levels can vary between 'undetectable' levels to values exceeding 2 – 3 million 'copies' / mm^3 of blood. Levels below 400 are considered 'undetectable'.

> **The viral load is the best indicator of the rapidity ('speed') of the development of immune-deficiency and AIDS. The higher the viral load, the sooner immune-deficiency is likely to develop.**
>
> **People with higher viral loads are also more likely to spread HIV via sex, pregnancy and breast feeding.**

The above is illustrated on page 76.

◆ Will everyone with HIV infection go on to develop AIDS?

It is not yet clear whether every HIV-infected person will progress to develop illness and AIDS. Approximately 80% of HIV-infected people will have developed AIDS within 12 years of acquiring the infection. On average, it takes about 8 years from HIV infection to AIDS. It seems likely that most HIV-infected people will eventually develop severe immune-deficiency and symptomatic disease, even if this takes 15 – 20 years. New therapy with anti-HIV drugs can alter the course of the disease (*see Chapter 5*).

HIV-infected people can be rapid or slow progressors.

Rapid progressors

- ◆ People who are rapid progressors usually develop immune-deficiency earlier, often within 5 – 7 years after infection.

- ◆ For some this may be as soon as 3 – 4 years.

Slow progressors

◆ Slow progressors generally remain well and active without any disease, and with very little or absent immune-deficiency.

◆ These individuals may remain well for 10 – 15 years or more.

Non-progressors

◆ A small percentage of infected people (usually about 5%) remain well and free of immune-deficiency.

◆ They may never progress to immune-deficiency and HIV-related illness.

The existing health status of an individual may influence how long it will take to develop immune-deficiency and symptomatic disease. Diseases like malnutrition, measles, tuberculosis, malaria etc. may have an independent immuno-depressive effect. This may alter the natural course of the HIV disease.

The various stages of HIV disease are discussed in more detail below.

> **Some patients may be rapid progressors to immune-deficiency and AIDS. Others may be slow progressors, and a very small and lucky proportion are non-progressors.**

 ## Early (Primary) HIV infection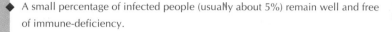

> **In the first 3 – 6 months after acquiring the HIV infection, there may be a short (1 – 2 weeks) sero-conversion illness which causes the following:**
>
> ◆ Fever, headache
> ◆ Tiredness, malaise, myalgia
> ◆ Rash
> ◆ Sore throat
> ◆ Muscle and joint pains
> ◆ Some swelling of the lymph glands
> ◆ Gastro-intestinal symptoms

This occurs at the time when the HIV antibody test usually converts from being **negative to positive**, so the clinical condition is referred to as the **sero-conversion illness**. Because the signs and symptoms are non-specific, the sero-conversion illness is often mistaken for a 'flu-like', viral illness or glandular fever. It often passes unnoticed by the patient.

The HIV antibody test usually becomes **positive** 4 – 6 weeks after infection (see page 41). Often, for the first 1 – 5 years or more, the HIV test may be the only indication that a person has HIV, with no other signs of illness.

> **In the first few years after HIV infection, the HIV antibody test may be the *only sign* of HIV infection.**

After the initial non-specific symptoms of HIV infection and sero-conversion, the patient usually remains well and asymptomatic. This is often called the **clinically latent or 'silent' phase** of HIV infection.

The HIV viral load may rise to high levels before the sero-conversion illness, and then drop to much lower levels thereafter. ART may be very effective if given in these early weeks of infection. It may reduce the viral load, and possibly offer the patient a better future.

The level that the viral load reaches at this stage of the disease is called the 'set point,' and ART can reduce this set point (*see diagram on page 76*). A lower set point is likely to result in a lowered viral burden (load) in the body, and a better outlook (prognosis). For this reason it is important to detect HIV infection early, and to commence ART before or during the primary HIV infection illness. This 'early detection' of HIV is missed in most patients. This is especially important after needlestick injuries, rape and other known risky sexual encounters. ART should be given for 9 – 12 months only for primary HIV infection.

Clinical latent or 'silent' infection – the asymptomatic phase

The HIV-infected person usually experiences a period of good health in which the virus remains clinically 'silent' or latent. The phase may last between 3 and 7 years (even up to 10 years). However, even though the infection is clinically 'silent', the virus is active in the body, usually causing progressive damage to the immune system. The person is able to spread the virus during this phase. The CD4 cell count will usually decrease by 40 – 80 cells / ml per year.

The asymptomatic phase is usually associated with a CD4 cell count between 500 and 800 cells / mm³ or even less (*see table on page 26*).

> **Even though the infection is clinically 'silent', the virus is active in the body and the person is able to spread the virus during this phase.**

Minor HIV-related symptoms
– the minor symptomatic phase

Between 3 and 7 years after infection, some individuals may develop 'minor' symptoms and signs secondary to the HIV infection.

These may include the following:

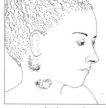

Lymphadenopathy

◆ Chronic swelling of the lymph nodes, which are commonly felt in the neck, axilla and below the jaw (often called '**persistent generalised lymphadenopathy**')

◆ Herpes zoster

◆ Occasional fevers

◆ Skin rashes, such as folliculitis, seborrhoeic dermatitis and chronic itchy skin

◆ Fungal nail infections

◆ Recurrent oral ulcerations (aphthous), angular stomatitis, cheilitis

◆ Recurrent upper respiratory tract infections

The minor symptomatic phase is usually associated with a CD4 cell count between 350 and 500 cells / mm³ (*see table on page 26*).

HIV-related disease
– the symptomatic phase

After about 5 – 8 years following HIV infection, the viral load tends to increase progressively, and the immune system continues to deteriorate and become immune-deficient *(see Chapter 6)*. Signs of more severe HIV-related disease begin to appear.

These signs and symptoms are usually due to overgrowth of some of the body's natural flora with fungal infection and reactivation of old infections (such as TB and herpes). They are also due to uncontrolled multiplication of HIV itself. Later, as the immune-deficiency progresses, more frequent and severe opportunistic infections occur. This stage of HIV disease was previously called 'AIDS-related complex' (ARC).

FROM HIV TO AIDS

The most common signs and symptoms of this stage of HIV-related disease are as follows:

- Oral or vaginal candida infection (thrush)
  - this is usually persistent and recurrent
- Hairy leukoplakia on the tongue (*see page 137*)
- Recurrent herpes simplex infection
  - 'cold sores' or genital herpes infection
- Herpes zoster (shingles)
- Acne-like bacterial skin infections
- Persistent and unexplained fevers and night sweats
- Skin rashes (*see page 137*)
- Generalised lymphadenopathy or shrinking of previously enlarged lymph nodes
- Persistent diarrhoea
- Weight loss (more than 10% of usual body weight)
- Reactivation of tuberculosis may also be associated with this stage of infection, especially in people from low socio-economic communities, where tuberculosis is common (endemic)

The symptomatic phase is usually associated with a CD4 cell count between 150 and 350 cells / mm³. The onset of the conditions associated with more advanced immune-deficiency are outlined later (*see table on page 26*).

> **The onset of oral / vaginal candidiasis (thrush) and recurrent herpes infection, such as herpes simplex (cold sores) or herpes zoster (shingles), are commonly the first clinical signs of advanced immune-deficiency.**

Severe HIV-related disease
– AIDS, the severe symptomatic phase

The symptomatic phase, described *on page 30*, usually progresses over the next year or 18 months into the fully developed AIDS phase of the disease.

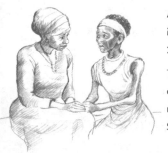

AIDS is almost always associated with a high HIV viral load and severe immune-deficiency. This usually coresponds to CD4 cell counts below 200 cell / mm³ and to a low lymphocyte count.

This allows the development of severe opportunistic infections, some cancers and HIV-related organ damage. These conditions are therefore referred to as '**AIDS defining' illnesses** and are listed in the WHO Staging System for HIV Infection and Disease *(on page 118)*.

◆ Symptoms of AIDS

Signs and symptoms of AIDS may differ from one patient to another and depending on which infection, cancer or organ is affected e.g.

- ◆ Herpes, seborrhoeic dermatitis, skin sepsis may present with a variety of **skin rashes and skin conditions**.
- ◆ Respiratory infection usually presents with persistent **cough, chest pain and fever**.
- ◆ Candidiasis presents with **oral and /or genital thrush**.
- ◆ Infection of the bowel will present with **ongoing diarrhoea**.
- ◆ Infection of the brain will present with **headache, fits and other neurological conditions**.
- ◆ Cancers, such as Kaposi's sarcoma, appear as **reddish, purple spots on the skin and mucous membranes** that increase in size and number. Lymphoma may present with **enlarged lymph nodes, liver or spleen**.
- ◆ People with AIDS usually experience severe **tiredness, fatigue and weakness**.
- ◆ Occasionally there may be some **memory and concentration loss**, and some people may eventually develop **severe mental deterioration and confusion**.

Manifestations of AIDS may include any of the conditions on *pages 30 – 31*. There may also be some of the following:

- ◆ Skin rashes
- ◆ Persistent, worsening cough and pneumonia
- ◆ Nausea, vomiting and diarrhoea (lasting more than 2 weeks)
- ◆ Peripheral neuropathy (e.g. pains, 'pins and needles' or numbness in the hands and feet)
- ◆ Persistent headache, convulsions and signs of meningitis, dementia
- ◆ Poor concentration, memory loss, confusion
- ◆ Wasting of the body's tissues and marked weight loss
- ◆ Difficulty and pain on swallowing (usually due to candidiasis of the throat and oesophagus)
- ◆ Retinitis and blindness (usually due to cytomegalovirus)
- ◆ Various cancers such as Kaposi's sarcoma, non-Hodgkin's lymphoma, ano-genital and liver (hepatitis B or C associated)
- ◆ It is now evident that many organ systems such as the heart, kidney and brain may be affected by HIV.

The presence of any serious opportunistic infection is a sign that the body is not coping immunologically.

The following table lists the common opportunistic infections and cancers associated with AIDS.

These conditions cause most of the symptoms on the previous page. *They will be described in more detail in later chapters.*

◆ **Bacteria**

 – *Mycobacterium tuberculosis* – lungs and other body organs, including the meninges .

 – Group B streptococcus – lungs (usually in children)

 – *Haemophilus influenzae* – lungs (usually in children)

 – Pneumococci – lung and blood stream

 – Salmonella – GIT and blood

 – Atypical mycobacterium – lung and other organs

◆ **Viruses**

 – Herpes simplex – skin and nervous system

 – Herpes zoster (shingles) – skin and nervous system

 – Cytomegalovirus – lungs, retina, brain, GIT and liver

◆ **Protozoa**

 – *Pneumocystis carinii* – lungs

 – Toxoplasmosis – meninges, brain and eye

 – Cryptosporidium – GIT and gall-bladder

◆ **Fungi**

 – Candida – mouth, oesophagus, intestinal tract, vagina, skin and nails

 – Cryptococcus – meninges and lungs

 – Histoplasmosis – lungs

◆ **Cancer**

 – Kaposi's sarcoma – skin, GIT

 – Lymphomas – non-Hodgkin's

 – Ano-genital (human papilloma virus)

 – Liver (associated with hepatitis B or C)

 – Multi-centre (Castleman's disease)

The following table lists common organs affected by opportunistic infections:

◆ **Blood stream**
Pneumococci
Salmonella

◆ **Bone marrow**
TB and other mycobacteria
Cytomegalovirus
Cryptococcus
Histoplasmosis

◆ **Eye (retina)**
Cytomegalovirus
Toxoplasmosis
Herpes zoster
HIV

◆ **Gall-bladder**
Cryptosporidium

◆ **Gastro-intestinal**
Salmonella
Cytomegalovirus
Cryptosporidium
Candida

◆ **Genital tract**
Candida

◆ **Kidney**
TB and other mycobacteria
Cytomegalovirus

◆ **Liver**
Cytomegalovirus

◆ **Nervous system / brain**
Mycobacterium tuberculosis
Cytomegalovirus
Herpes simplex and zoster
Toxoplasmosis
Cryptococcus

◆ **Oral / oesophageal infection**
Herpes simplex

◆ **Respiratory infection**
Mycobacterium tuberculosis
Group B streptococcus
Haemophilus influenzae
Atypical mycobacterium
Pneumococci
Cryptococcus
Cytomegalovirus
Pneumocystis carinii
Histoplasmosis

◆ **Skin**
Herpes simplex and zoster
Candida

From the above it is clear that AIDS is not a single disease with a characteristic set of signs and symptoms.

It consists of, and may present with, a variety of signs and symptoms, depending on which specific infection or cancer is present. It also depends on which organ is mostly affected.

These conditions usually occur late in the course of HIV infection and arise due to the deteriorating immune-deficiency.

The WHO Staging System for HIV Infection and Disease and the CDC case definition of AIDS provide a more complete outline of HIV/AIDS-related conditions (see pages 118 – 120).

People with AIDS often go through stages of being very sick with severe disease, to being reasonably well again (usually due to treatment). However infections tend to re-occur and become more frequent. The body becomes progressively weaker with repeated infection, with the multiplication of HIV, and possibly due to the development of various cancers. Death usually occurs 6 months to 3 years after developing signs of AIDS.

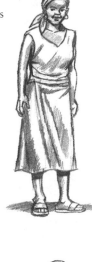

The availability of ART and the prevention and treatment of the opportunistic infections, such as TB, *Pneumocystis carinii*, candidiasis etc., can modify the progress of the disease. Modern ART can significantly prolong the patient's wellness and reduce the severity and frequency of opportunistic infections.

HIV/AIDS has a very variable clinical course. There are very few rules.

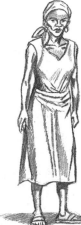

- Some patients progress rapidly and others more slowly.
- Serious and severe opportunistic infections can appear at a variety of different clinical and immune levels.
- Some patients may suddenly deteriorate and progress very rapidly to severe illness and death.
- Some may have a slow and gentle decline, and others an unpredictable course of long periods of health with occasional periods of sickness.
- Some may remain very well for many years and then suddenly deteriorate.
- Some may never get ill.
- Some may get repeated opportunistic infections with many different conditions.
- Some may only suffer from a few of the common opportunistic illnesses.
- Some patients can get reasonably well after being very sick.
- Some patients tolerate ART well, but others do not.
- ART may be very effective in some patients and less so in others.

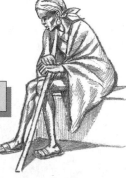

The unexpected can and sometimes does happen.

The HIV antibody test and issues relevant to the test are discussed in the next chapter.

FROM HIV TO AIDS

Additional notes for new developments

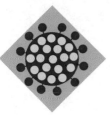

Chapter 4

HIV TESTING AND PRE-TEST/POST-TEST COUNSELLING

Diagnosing HIV infection

HIV antibody tests

Pre-test and post-test counselling

Diagnosing HIV infection

HIV infection in adults is often 'silent', and the patient usually remains symptom-free for many years (3 – 10 years). In children the signs and symptoms may appear earlier, and the signs and symptoms of AIDS may appear in the first few months or within a year or two (*see Chapter 8*).

In many patients the only evidence of HIV infection is a positive HIV test. For other patients signs and symptoms of AIDS or immune-deficiency make the chances of HIV infection more probable.

HIV testing is normally done if:

◆ There are clinical signs suggestive of HIV infection (*see pages 63 and 103*).

◆ There are other clinical indications, such as testing during ante-natal care
   – or if there are associated diseases such as tuberculosis (TB) or sexually transmitted infections (STIs).

◆ There are other purposes, e.g. as part of the blood-donating screening process, post-needlestick injuries etc.

HIV testing should be done in a proper and ethical manner

◆ Before HIV testing is done, pre- and post-test counselling must always be offered to the patient.

◆ It is important for the patient to understand:
   – the reason for the HIV test
   – the nature of the test
   – the meaning of an HIV positive and negative result
   – the possible psycho-social implications of the result
   – the follow-up plan

◆ The patient must consent to have the test. This should be on the basis of correct and accurate information ('informed consent').

◆ Testing should never be done without consent or against the patient's wishes.

Pre- and post-test counselling is discussed in detail in Chapter 13.

◆ HIV is usually diagnosed by the following methods

An HIV antibody test

HIV antibody tests are usually done on blood (serum). However it is possible to detect antibodies in other body fluids such as saliva and urine. It must be remembered that this is an **HIV antibody test**, and it does not detect the actual HIV virus. Antibody tests detect the presence of *antibodies* which is the body's response to the HIV infection.

Antibody tests are usually detected by the ELISA or a Western blot method of testing. These tests are usually done in the laboratory. However rapid 'bedside' tests are also available (*see page 46*). The Western Blot test is the more complex and expensive test.

HIV antibody tests are the most common form of testing and are widely available and not expensive. Antibody tests usually become positive approximately 6 weeks after infection.

> **An individual who has tested positive for HIV antibodies is called 'HIV positive'. Adults usually test HIV positive approximately 6 weeks after being infected with HIV.**

HIV p24 antigen and HIV PCR tests

Antigen tests detect the actual HIV virus. The tests pick up actual components of the HIV virus. Antigen tests are commonly known as HIV p24 antigen tests. The p24 antigen test is often useful in certain clinical situations, but it lacks sensitivity.

An **HIV PCR RNA** (polymerase chain reaction) test can also be done. This can be a qualitative test (i.e. negative or positive result), or a quantitative test (i.e. the **number** of viral RNA particles / ml of blood). This is also called the **HIV viral load test** (*see also page 74, Chapter 5*).

These tests are not widely available and usually need sophisticated laboratories and are expensive. Antigen tests become positive within the first 10 – 14 days after infection, and are most valuable for diagnosing infection early and for detection of newborn infection.

A negative test in the first 2 weeks after infection may be false negative and should be repeated. In babies the tests are more reliable from approximately 1 month after birth.

Signs and symptoms of immune-deficiency and AIDS

It is also possible to diagnose HIV infection by detecting very specific HIV-related conditions such a Kaposi's sarcoma (in < 65 year olds), PCP pneumonia and other 'AIDS-defining or indicator' conditions (*see page 104*).

The next section will discuss the HIV tests in more detail.

HIV antibody tests

After HIV infection it usually takes approximately 6 weeks before the test is able to detect the HIV antibodies. The graph below illustrates the development of antibodies, the conversion from HIV negative to HIV positive i.e. the sero-conversion, and the window period.

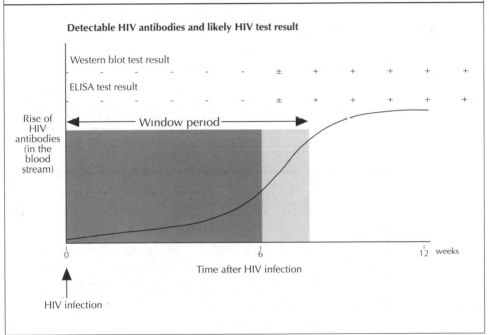

THE DEVELOPMENT OF HIV ANTIBODIES IN THE BLOOD AFTER HIV INFECTION

Detectable HIV antibodies and likely HIV test result

Western blot test result

| - | - | - | - | - | ± | + | + | + | + | + |

ELISA test result

| - | - | - | - | - | ± | + | + | + | + |

Rise of HIV antibodies (in the blood stream)

Window period

0   6   12   weeks

Time after HIV infection

HIV infection

◆ The window period

Antibodies are usually detected after about 6 weeks following HIV infection. Some individuals may need 12 weeks, and very few may need 6 – 12 months before their HIV test becomes positive. This period, after HIV infection and before the test becomes positive, is called the **window period**.

Even though the test is negative early after infection, the person is able to pass on the virus to others during this 'window' period.

If a test result is negative, and you suspect that the test has been done too early after a possible infection, you must advise the person to have a repeat test. This repeat test should be done at least 12 weeks after any likely risk of infection (*see also HIV antigen / PCR tests on page 46*).

The 'window' period is the stage during which:
- **The person is HIV-infected**
- **The HIV antibody test is still negative**
- **The virus can be passed on to others.**

The p24 antigen and the HIV PCR tests are usually positive during the window period.

◆ The ELISA antibody test

- The HIV ELISA antibody test is the most popular and commonly used test. It is sufficient to make a diagnosis of HIV infection.

- HIV ELISA tests are widely available and reasonably cheap.

- The ELISA tests are also available as rapid tests. These 'rapid' tests do not need a laboratory and can be done in the consulting rooms / clinic. Rapid tests are generally reasonably reliable. However any positive rapid HIV antibody test should be confirmed by a formal laboratory test. *Rapid testing is discussed on page 46.*

- The ELISA tests are excellent screening tests.

- ELISA tests are very sensitive i.e. if a person is HIV positive, then the test is very reliable in actually testing positive. Most tests have a 99+% sensitivity with very few false negative results. Occasionally they may test positively when the person is not truly HIV infected i.e. a false positive. For this reason an HIV positive test should always be confirmed with another test.

Confirming an initial ELISA HIV positive antibody test

- In countries where there is high HIV prevalence (> 10%), the likelihood of a false positive result is much less when compared with countries with a lower HIV prevalence. In South Africa 2 positive HIV ELISA tests are now considered adequate evidence of a true HIV infection (*see the following page*).

- Most HIV ELISA antibody tests are highly sensitive. However there is a very low probability of the test being falsely positive (usually less than 1%). For this reason, a patient should have at least 2 positive antibody tests.

A single HIV-positive ELISA test should be confirmed as follows:

◆ Another ELISA test should be done on the same specimen, preferably with a different testing method / design (the laboratory would know which method to use).

◆ In outlying or remote areas, or where resources are limited, a rapid HIV test could also be used to confirm the result.

Special circumstances

In special circumstances, e.g. a newborn baby, or an indeterminate ELISA test, confirmation can also be done with:

◆ A Western Blot (WB) antibody test (for indeterminate ELISA tests)

◆ An HIV p24 antigen or an HIV PCR test

Note: The WB and the PCR are more costly and less widely available. They should not be used routinely as confirmatory tests.

> It may not be necessary to confirm a positive HIV test antibody result if there are other indicators of HIV infection such as:
>
> – obvious signs and symptoms of immune-deficiency / AIDS / HIV-related opportunistic infections
> – and / or laboratory evidence of immune-deficiency and there is a low CD4 cell count (*see pages 77 – 78*).

◆ Interpreting an HIV antibody test

An HIV 'positive' (or 'reactive') test result

The HIV positive test result means:

◆ There is definite HIV infection if there are other obvious signs of immune-deficiency.

◆ There is likely HIV infection and a confirmatory test should be done (see above).

◆ The person is able to spread the HIV during sex, through his / her blood, or during pregnancy, childbirth and breast feeding.

Very rarely it may be a 'false positive' result.

> **An HIV test does not tell whether you have AIDS.**
> **It only determines whether you have been infected with the HIV virus.**

The HIV positive test result does NOT:

◆ Mean that the person has developed the AIDS stage of the HIV disease.

◆ Mean that the person will definitely develop AIDS. However, most HIV positive people (95%) will develop AIDS within 7 – 10 years from the time of the infection (not from the time of the test!).

◆ Reveal the stage of the disease.

◆ Determine when the person acquired the HIV infection.

An HIV negative (non 'reactive') test result

The HIV negative test result means:

◆ The patient does not have HIV infection, unless the test is done in the window period.

◆ It may be falsely negative if the test is done within the first 6 – 12 weeks after HIV infection. If the test is done within the first 6 – 12 weeks after possible HIV exposure, then the test should be repeated after a total period of 12 weeks after the possible HIV exposure.

Indeterminate test results

◆ Sometimes an indeterminate result is given. This means the test is not clear either way. It should then be repeated in the near future or a Western Blot antibody test or HIV antigen or PCR test should be done if possible.

◆ Occasionally the test may be falsely negative. In other words the test is negative, but the person is actually HIV-infected. This may be due to the 'window period' or to some technical problem. On rare occasions it may be due to very severe immune-deficiency.

◆ Sometimes the laboratory or the health care worker may make a mistake in labelling or reporting the result (this is very uncommon but it can happen).

◆ When to re-test a person who has an HIV negative test result

One way to decide whether you should test the patient again is by finding out if the patient or his/her sexual partner has been at risk of acquiring HIV in the 6 – 12 weeks before the test was done.

Ask if there has been any risky sexual activity in the 6 – 12 weeks before having the test.

Risky sexual activity may include:

- Having sex without a condom with a new partner
- Having sex with more than one partner without using a condom every time
- Having sex with a sex worker (prostitute) without using a condom

Other risk factors that are important include:

- Any sexually transmitted infection in the past 3 months
- Any sharing of needles and syringes or blood transfusions in the past 3 months

Also make sure you ask about the patient's sexual partner. Has the sexual partner been at risk over the past 3 months?

Risky sexual activity

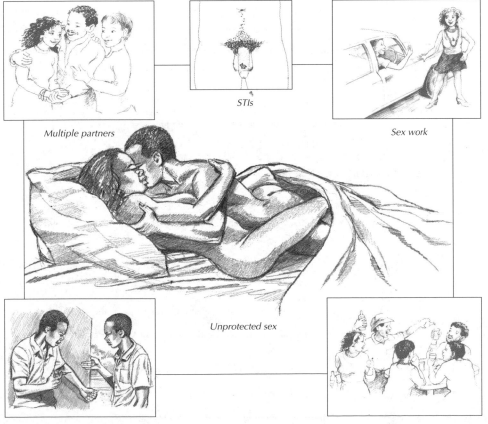

Multiple partners

STIs

Sex work

Unprotected sex

Sharing needles during intravenous drug use

Alcohol and sex

If you feel that there is a possibility of HIV infection in the past 12 weeks, then you should recommend another test in 2 – 3 months time. During this period you should advise the use of condoms until the result of the test is known.

A person with a negative result must not think that he/she is immune to (safe from) HIV infection.

An HIV test result needs careful interpretation.

◆ HIV antigen and PCR tests

In recent years HIV antigen and HIV PCR tests have become more available in some of the larger centres. These test for the actual HIV virus. They are commonly known as the P24 HIV antigen test and the HIV RNA PCR test.

◆ Antigen / PCR tests usually become positive within 7 – 14 days after HIV infection.

◆ The p24 antigen test is more likely to be positive around the sero-conversion period *(see page 28)* and in the more advanced stages of the disease.

◆ Antigen and PCR tests are expensive and usually not necessary for HIV diagnosis. There is also a higher false positive rate in the very early stage of HIV infection.

◆ These tests are usually only indicated if:
  – it is necessary to know the HIV status very early (i.e. within the window period)
  – the antibody tests are indeterminate
  – in special circumstances, such as in a newborn baby, post rape etc.

◆ Rapid HIV tests

Rapid HIV testing refers to a HIV antibody testing which usually can be performed more quickly (5 – 30 minutes) than the standard laboratory-based tests.

◆ Many of these tests can be done without the need for a formal laboratory, often 'at the bed side'.

◆ These tests are relatively easy to use, and cheaper than standard laboratory tests.

◆ The tests can usually be operated and read by non-laboratory personnel such as clinical doctors and nurses. Some are even being marketed to the lay public for 'self testing' purposes, but this practice is not advised.

◆ The tests can be incorrect if the testing protocol is not followed exactly.

◆ Many of these tests are able to provide a result within 10 – 30 minutes.

Sensitivities and specificities

The sensitivities (accuracy in detecting HIV positivity) and the specificities (accuracy in detecting HIV negativity) of the good quality, rapid, short incubation tests are similar to those of the standard laboratory-based ELISA tests (some of the rapid tests are of poor quality, and users should check this out before using various tests).

However they are more likely to miss sero-conversion, or late stage HIV infection, because they are often less able to detect low levels of antibody.

A confirmatory, laboratory-based ELISA HIV test should be done on all rapid HIV positive reactive test results.

The accuracy and reliability of rapid tests are dependent on the test being performed properly and the result read accurately. Many of the tests require a comparison or matching of the colour of the final outcome of the reagents or of agglutination of the reagents. It is critical that these colour readings are done accurately. It is also important to perform proper quality controls on the tests, and to check shelf-life (expiry date), the controls and the exact time needed etc.

> **The accuracy and reliability of rapid tests are dependent on the test being performed properly and the result read accurately.**

Role for rapid HIV testing

Rapid diagnosis of HIV infection

- In some clinical situations, it may be important to have a rapid HIV diagnosis so that immediate appropriate therapy can be provided.

Diagnosing HIV infection in areas without local, adequate, diagnostic laboratories or facilities

- In some isolated areas, diagnostic laboratories are often far away. This means there is inconvenience and delay in submitting specimens or obtaining results.

- Rapid testing in these situations can help with a early diagnosis e.g.
    - in a rural hospital which does not have the necessary laboratory resources
    - in isolated communities being served only by a clinic or a few clinical health care personnel

Clinical screening

- In various clinical situations it may be important to know the HIV status of the patient. Rapid testing may be appropriate and more cost effective when compared with formal laboratory testing e.g.
    - antenatal testing
    - patients with STIs or TB
    - patients with clinical signs that may suggest HIV infection

- A formal laboratory confirmation test should be done on all positive results.

Biohazardous injuries (needlestick injuries) or post-sexual abuse

◆ The recommended management of occupationally acquired HIV exposure (e.g. needlestick injuries) includes the immediate use of ART for post-exposure prophylaxis (*see pages 320 – 327*).

◆ Rapid diagnosis (or exclusion) of HIV infection in the source patient or in the specimen from which the injury occurred (e.g. in a laboratory worker) will help to decide whether ART should be commenced.

◆ ART should be commenced immediately after such injuries
  – the rapid test will facilitate much earlier institution of ART in these circumstances

◆ This may also apply to a post-rape situation.

Epidemiological surveillance and other screening

◆ Rapid HIV tests are useful for epidemiological purposes, such as for unlinked surveillance of HIV.

HIV testing where follow-up is unlikely or difficult

◆ In some situations, especially in deep rural areas, returning for specific HIV test results may be difficult or costly for the patient.

◆ A rapid test offers the opportunity for on-site testing and being able to give the results at the same time. Confirmation of a rapid test in these settings can be done with a second *different rapid test*.

Some important issues to consider when doing rapid HIV testing

Implications for health care workers and patients

◆ Rapid tests should not imply a rapid management of the patient, nor should they imply that results are necessarily given in a more rapid process.

◆ Rapid testing can place undue pressure on the health care worker and on the patient. Psycho-social management of the patient may be threatened by the rapid testing process.

Reading and interpreting the rapid test

◆ Rapid tests are not necessarily easy to do or easy to interpret.

◆ *Non-laboratory staff doing such tests may not have the necessary experience or knowledge of how to do the test correctly.*

◆ Adequate training and experience is necessary before health care workers use these tests.

Confirmation tests

◆ A confirmatory formal laboratory test should be offered to all patients who test positive on the rapid test
  – confirmatory tests are not generally necessary if the test result is negative.

◆ It may not be necessary to do a confirmatory test if there are signs of immune-deficiency (oral thrush, Kaposi's sarcoma, PCP etc.)

Counselling

Rapid HIV testing must be carried out according to the proper and ethical standards as for any other HIV test.

There must be:

◆ Pre- and post-test counselling

◆ Informed consent

◆ Privacy, confidentiality and the right to refuse to have the test

A rapid test does not mean that you can rapidly bypass any proper process for doing HIV tests. There is major concern that informed consent may not always be obtained or that proper pre- and post-test counselling will not be offered. Rapid tests highlight the importance of maintaining the highest ethical standards surrounding HIV testing.

Counsellors providing POSITIVE test results should do the following:

◆ They should explain the meaning of the reactive screening test result
  – they should explain the likelihood of HIV infection
  – they should also explain that a confirmatory test will determine with more certainty whether the individual is HIV positive or not.

◆ Disclosure of any test result to partners by the HIV-positive person needs to be done with caution
  – it is recommended that partners should only be notified by the patient after the result has been confirmed by a standard HIV laboratory test.

◆ The patient should be advised to take precautions to prevent HIV transmission i.e. to act as if he / she is HIV infected and to use condoms
  – this should be carried out until the result has been formally confirmed.

◆ The issues such as follow-up, partner disclosure, confirming the test result, referral to care centres, cost and role of ART etc. should be discussed during the pre-test counselling session.

◆ Arrange for a formal laboratory confirmatory test such as an ELISA
  – arrange a return visit to get the confirmatory result.

◆ Discuss whether and how to disclose the result of the rapid test to partners and other persons important to the patient (prior to a confirmed result)
  – give options for support and psycho-social referral.

◆ HIV testing needs to be done with much care and consideration

AIDS is a very serious disease and sadly there is much misconception, discrimination and prejudice against HIV-infected people. A positive HIV result often causes a crisis that can dramatically change the person's life. This may have serious implications for the future.

An HIV-positive person may have to make some very important decisions and changes to his/her life, such as:

- ◆ It may mean changing sexual habits to avoid passing the virus to his / her sexual partner (*see page 96*).

- ◆ Considering the option of ART, which will involve cost, adhering to drug regimens, health care monitoring etc.

- ◆ It may also be difficult to adjust to the idea that his / her life may be significantly shortened or a life requiring constant medical support.

- ◆ He / she may have a fear of developing serious disease.

- ◆ He / she may not understand the meaning of the test. The person may wrongly think he / she is going to die soon.

- ◆ Decisions about having children need to be carefully considered. This is because of the risk of infecting the unborn child, and the possibility of the parent/s dying before the child has grown up. This is especially true if the drugs to prevent mother to child transmission are unavailable.

There may be many reasons that require counselling:

- ◆ Many relationships have broken up due to one partner being HIV positive.

- ◆ People have lost their jobs and have even been rejected by their friends and family.

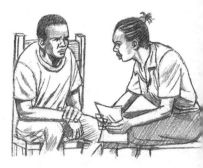

- ◆ Feelings of depression, anger and guilt may result. Some people have even committed suicide after receiving their HIV test results.

This means that everyone who has an HIV test must be properly counselled about the test **before** the test is done (a **pre-test counsel** or **interview**).

It is equally important to carefully counsel a person **after** the test (a **post-test counsel** or **interview**).

These are discussed in the section following.

Pre-test and post-test counselling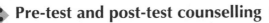

◆ Counselling before the test

Reasons for pre-test counselling include:

◆ To ensure that the person understands the basic facts about HIV infection and AIDS

◆ To assist the patient in understanding the test and what the results mean and to prepare him / her to receive this result

◆ To consider and explore what he / she might do if the test is positive or negative

◆ To explore potential support from loved ones, family, friends etc.

◆ To understand that if he / she is HIV positive, there is medical care e.g. ART and monitoring which can help to keep him / her healthier for longer (*see Chapter 5*)

◆ To ensure that the person has confidence in the confidentiality of the test result i.e. that it will be kept private

◆ To advise on safer sexual practices (*see page 96*)

◆ To enable the person to make an informed decision whether to take the test or not

◆ To make an assessment of risk of possible HIV infection

Some of the most important issues which you should explore and discuss BEFORE an HIV test is done:

◆ Does the patient understand the basic information about AIDS and HIV infection? Explain these and clear up any misunderstandings.

◆ Does the patient understand what the test is and what a positive or negative result would mean? Remember it is an antibody test and does not tell whether you have the AIDS phase of the disease.

◆ Explore why he / she wants the test, or explain why you have suggested the test, and what benefits there are in knowing HIV status. Has he / she been at risk for acquiring HIV infection?

◆ It is also important to discuss how the patient thinks he / she might feel and react if the test is positive. How would he / she tell the news of the result to the sexual partner? If the result is positive, the sexual partner may also need a test.

◆ It is best if he / she thinks carefully about who to tell the result to. Employers, friends, and even some family members may not keep the result to themselves. Many people have lost their jobs, friends and lovers after telling them the positive result.

◆ Does he / she know how to prevent the spread of HIV infection? Does he / she know how to have sex in a safer way? Can he / she get condoms or do you need to provide them? Does he / she know how to use them correctly? You may need to explain in detail about the importance of practising safer sex from now onwards. Remember this may be the last time you will see the patient (*see page 96*).

◆ Explain when and how he / she can get the result. HIV results should be given to patients in person and in privacy. The result must be kept confidential.

◆ Let him / her know that you understand the difficulty and anxieties involved in having an HIV test. Let him / her know that you, or another health worker, will be available to give the result. Tell him / her that it will be kept confidential and that there will be ongoing support and advice if needed.

◆ After exploring the above issues, it is important finally to ask if he / she still wants to undergo the test, or would he / she like to think about it a little longer? In this way he / she will be able to give informed consent to have the test.

It is best for the client to make the final decision and choice to have the test or not.

◆ Counselling after the test

Reasons for post-test counselling include:

◆ It is often difficult for a person to accept and believe that he / she has HIV infection merely on the basis of an HIV positive test result. Counselling is often needed to help convince the patient about the reality of the situation.

◆ To ensure the person understands the meaning of the result.

◆ To help the person cope with the result, especially in the days or weeks to follow (if the result is positive).

◆ To make a follow-up plan for the ongoing medical and supportive care of the person if he / she is HIV positive.

◆ To ensure that the person is aware of the dangers of spreading HIV (if the result is positive) or of preventing infection (if the result is negative). Information on safer sexual practices should also be given (*see page 96*).

◆ To understand the need for careful consideration about having children, if HIV positive (*see page 217*).

◆ To explain the need for re-testing if he/she is considered to be in the 'window' period.

Remember to carefully counsel those whose HIV result is negative, to avoid further risk of HIV infection.

Some of the most important issues to discuss AFTER giving the HIV test result.

It is usually best to give the result as soon as possible without any unnecessary delay.

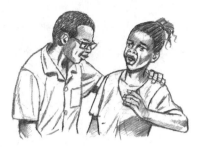

Results must be given in a private and confidential manner.

Remember the patient is most likely to be very anxious and will be concerned about the result. Allow him / her time to think about it. Whether it is positive or negative, you must check that he / she understands the meaning of the result, and what the implications are. He / she may need to return to clear up misunderstandings or to hear some of the details again.

If the HIV test result is positive:

♦ Give the patient time to express his / her feelings and fears, and encourage him / her to talk. He / she may experience many different feelings, such as anger, guilt, sadness, anxiety, fear, confusion or disbelief. He / she may become emotionally 'shocked', or be unclear or confused about what to do next. These are all normal and expected responses. Give him / her the opportunity to feel them and express them.

♦ Reassure that he / she will not be abandoned (left alone). Make it clear that he / she will be supported and guided as to what to do next. Explain that coming to terms with the result is a process that needs some time.

♦ Try not to overload him / her with information and advice all at once. He / she needs to understand that there is much that can be offered by the health service to treat and manage an HIV-positive person. Let him / her know that you, or other co-workers, are available to provide ongoing support and care.

♦ ART is now an option for some HIV-positive people. However, there are issues around accessibility to this care, cost, adherence to therapy, regular monitoring, etc.

♦ He / she should understand the importance of practising safer sex, and the need to protect sexual partners from infection. He / she may need a supply of condoms.

♦ He / she may need convincing that an HIV positive result really means that there is HIV infection.

Condoms

♦ In a woman it is even more important for her to approach her sexual partner very carefully. The male partner may becomes aggressive and violent when he learns that his wife or girlfriend is HIV positive. He may even walk out on her and leave her destitute. The woman needs to think very carefully about what she should do.

◆ The patient must also be aware that he / she must not donate blood for transfusion or share a syringe, needle or razor blade with anyone else.

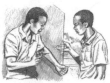

Sharing syringes

◆ You will need to discuss to whom he / she should tell the result and when to do so. Also discuss the possibility that he / she may be rejected by the partner, family etc.

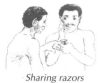

◆ You may need to make another time to discuss this and other questions and problems.

Sharing razors

Before leaving, make a time in the near future to meet again to discuss feelings and understanding of the situation. You will need to plan a follow-up care and management programme. He / she may want to bring the partner or another family member or trusted friend to this meeting.

If the HIV test result is negative:

◆ Check with the patient whether he / she understands the meaning of a negative result.

◆ If you feel he / she has had risk of exposure to infection in the 12 weeks before having the test (*see page 45*), then you may want to advise him / her to have another test in 6 – 12 months' time. Remember there is a 'window' period where a person is HIV-infected but the test is falsely negative.

◆ Discuss the importance of him / her remaining HIV negative. This means knowing how he / she could become infected in the future. The necessary precautions to prevent further infection will need to be taken (*see page 96*).

◆ You may need to counsel him / her about safer sexual practices. He / she must appreciate the seriousness of HIV infection and make a decision to practise sex in a safer way. It might be useful to explore why it has been difficult for him / her to practise safer sex.

◆ He / she also needs to understand the connection between other sexually transmitted diseases (STIs) and AIDS, and the importance of having the STI treated.

The primary care of people with HIV infection is discussed in the next chapter.

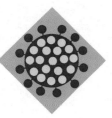

Chapter 5

PRIMARY CARE FOR EARLY (ASYMPTOMATIC) HIV INFECTION

The health worker/patient relationship

The first consultation

Establishing (confirming) the diagnosis and time
of HIV infection

Clinical assessment

Monitoring the HIV and immune status, and other investigations

Managing medical problems

Anti-retroviral therapy (ART)

Preventing opportunistic infections

Advice on self care, safer sexual practices
and a 'wellness' programme

Support, counselling and referral

This chapter will outline the management of a person with HIV in the earlier part of the disease. The relatively asymptomatic phase is discussed, before the development of major signs and symptoms and severe opportunistic infection etc.

The health worker / patient relationship

◆ The patient with HIV infection has an uncertain future

◆ It is often uncertain when HIV infection first occurred.

◆ It is uncertain for how long he / she will remain asymptomatic and well.

◆ If symptoms do develop, it is uncertain what exactly these symptoms will be.

◆ It is uncertain whether he / she will go on to develop AIDS and when this will occur.

◆ The patient's response to ART, and for how long the drugs will be effective may also be uncertain.

◆ When someone develops AIDS, it is uncertain how long he / she will live.

◆ In pregnancy it is uncertain whether the newborn will be infected (*see page 211*).

There are many other uncertainties.

> **Living with uncertainty is one of the most difficult problems for people with HIV/AIDS.**

◆ There is the need for a supportive health worker / patient relationship

◆ For the above reasons, it is important for the health worker and the HIV-positive person to establish a good, trusting, open and hopeful relationship.

◆ Continual support, encouragement and counselling is needed.

◆ The health worker must promote the involvement and participation of the patient in the management and therapeutic decisions.

Both patient and health worker must be on the look-out for the appearance of any unusual signs or symptoms. If detected early, it is usually possible to effectively manage most of the medical problems before serious disease has set in. A growing number of life-threatening opportunistic infections can also be treated if detected early.

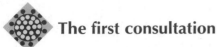

The first consultation

◆ The health care worker

Develop a trusting and caring relationship

People with HIV/AIDS have unique difficulties. They have a physical disease and they also have to cope with the stigma associated with HIV infection. There are many emotional and psychological issues as well.

Sometimes the health care worker is the only 'safe' person in whom the patient can confide. It is important to facilitate a good relationship with the patient at the first visit. You often need to be the health carer and the counsellor.

The health care provider should try to be:

◆ Warm and friendly

◆ Understanding of the difficulties of HIV infection

◆ Open to listening to the patient's issues

◆ Interested in the patient's life situation – job, family, partners, economic situation, etc.

◆ Non-judgemental

◆ As easily available or contactable as possible

◆ Able to empathise with the patient's burden

The above will encourage the patient to return for follow-up, comply with treatment, and take steps to live a healthier lifestyle.

◆ The management of a patient with asymptomatic or early stage HIV infection

◆ Confirm the diagnosis of HIV infection

◆ Encourage regular physical check-ups

◆ Monitor the HIV and the immune status

◆ Consider anti-retroviral therapy (ART)

◆ Prevent and treat opportunistic infection and disease

◆ Give advice on self care, wellness and safer sexual practices

◆ Support and counsel and keep hope alive

These are discussed on the following pages.

Establishing (confirming) the diagnosis and time of HIV infection

◆ Be sure of the HIV infection

To be sure of HIV infection, it is best to have more than one HIV positive result. In areas where the HIV infection is common, it is sufficient to have two positive ELISA HIV antibody tests using two different test methods on the same specimen (*see Chapter 4*).

Remember it is possible occasionally to have a false positive result, so two tests should be done. We no longer need the Western blot test for confirmation. It is an unnecessary expense in areas where infection rates are relatively high.

HIV RNA PCR testing can be used if necessary (*see page 40*).

The following is a guide to what would be acceptable as a diagnosis of HIV infection:

- ◆ Two ELISA laboratory-based tests on separate specimens or utilising separate test methods.

- ◆ One HIV-positive rapid HIV test and one positive laboratory ELISA test.

- ◆ One HIV-positive ELISA test and evidence of immune-deficiency (a low CD4 cell count).

- ◆ In very low-resourced areas, only one test may be affordable. Ideally in this situation, signs of immune-deficiency (*see page 102*) would help to confirm the likelihood of a true HIV infection, i.e. a positive HIV test in the presence of clear signs of immune-deficiency.

- ◆ One positive ELISA test and any AIDS-defining condition (*see page 43*).

- ◆ If there is any doubt of HIV infection, or if the antibody test is 'indeterminate', then a P24 HIV antigen test or an HIV RNA PCR is recommended (*see Chapter 4*).

◆ Try to establish the time of the HIV infection

Try to work out when the infection may have first occurred. Although this is often not possible, this knowledge may help to get an idea of the expected outlook of the patient. It is sometimes possible to isolate one or more possible risky sexual encounters in the past. They may give an indication of the time when the infection first occurred.

◆ There may be a past history of rape in an otherwise 'safe' sexual history.

◆ There may have been only one previous sexual partner and the relationship ended on a known date.

◆ There may have been an isolated sexual 'affair' outside of the usual or married partner.

◆ The patient may have visited a sex worker and had unprotected sex at a particular time.

◆ The patient may have had a blood transfusion in a country where the blood is not thoroughly tested.

◆ There may have been risky activity such as intravenous drug use, group ritual circumcision, group sexual encounters, etc.

◆ Any of the above may have occurred in the regular sexual partner.

◆ It is often impossible to establish when infection first occurred.

You may need to ask similar questions about the sexual partner

It is important to establish if the sexual partner has had an HIV test and whether he / she is HIV positive. The patient may have got the HIV **from** the partner or may have spread the HIV **to** the partner.

Occasionally it may be possible to get a history of the **sero-conversion illness** (primary HIV infection) associated with early HIV infection *(see page 28)*. This causes a short period (7 – 14 days) of symptoms, such as fever, lymphadenopathy, sore throat, muscle aches and joint pains.

Next you need to get an idea of the stage of the infection, and a baseline clinical and physical condition. It is also important to determine the HIV and the immune status.

Managing people with HIV/AIDS is both an 'art' and a 'science'. It is important to get to know the patient well, and to follow clinical and laboratory events carefully. There are guides and recommendations for various medical interventions. The clinician, however, will also need to develop a 'feel' about the patient, how his / her body is coping with the virus and with immune damage, and when best to intervene.

Clinical assessment

◆ The initial and ongoing clinical assessment sets out to do the following:

- ◆ It keeps a check on the physical, psychological and emotional condition.
- ◆ It detects and treats any new medical conditions early.
- ◆ It assesses the immune status.
- ◆ It assesses the HIV status.
- ◆ It makes clinical decisions to commence prevention (prophylaxis) therapy and ART.
- ◆ It assesses the social and economic circumstances of the patient.

Follow-ups

Check-ups should be done at relevant intervals. If the patient is well, asymptomatic and coping adequately, then the follow-ups may only be needed every 4 – 6 months.

If symptoms of the disease appear, or if prophylaxis therapy and / or ART has commenced, then the patient should be seen more often i.e. 2 – 3 monthly. If the patient is ill or in an advanced stage of the disease, he / she should be seen every 1 – 4 weeks.

> Symptoms of HIV disease usually appear 3 – 7 years after the first infection. It may even take up to 10 years. Regular monitoring can help identify and treat problems early which in turn will promote well-being.

◆ At the first visit and at each follow-up visit you should do the following:

- ◆ Take a careful history.
- ◆ Check and record the body weight.
- ◆ Examine specific areas thoroughly such as:
  - Skin
  - Mouth and teeth
  - Lymph nodes
  - Eyes
  - Genitals
  - Respiratory system
  - Abdomen
- ◆ Do a simple neurological assessment.
- ◆ Do a brief general examination.
- ◆ Do baseline tests / investigations.

◆ Take a careful history

It is important to take a careful, detailed history from the patient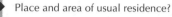

◆ The importance of trying to establish when the infection first occurred was discussed on *page 60.*

◆ You should also know the social and economic status / situation of the patient.

The following are some important questions concerning the social status of the patient

◆ Place and area of usual residence?

◆ Marital status and sexual partners?

◆ Family, children, pregnant wife?

◆ Employment and income?

◆ Social support?

◆ Access to health care, transport etc?

◆ Has the sexual partner also been tested and informed?

◆ Is the patient able to access and afford the ARV drugs on an ongoing basis?

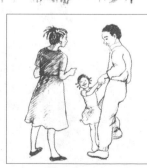

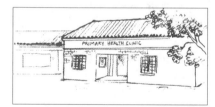

Access to health care and ART?

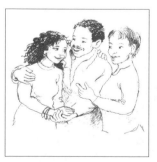

Multiple sexual habits?

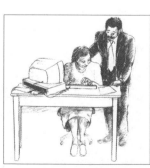

Employment?

Family situation?

Clinical features indicating early opportunistic infections

In addition, you should enquire about clinical features which may indicate early opportunistic infections, cancers or other conditions common in HIV-positive people.

◆ **Weight loss / anorexia (loss of appetite)**
Chronic infection, TB, diarrhoea, HIV infection, chronic chest infection, malignancy

◆ **Fever**
This may occur at night (e.g. tuberculosis, *Pneumocystis carinii*, HIV, septicaemia)

◆ **Respiratory problems**
Coughing, shortness of breath, chest pains (e.g. TB, *Pneumocystis carinii*, acute bacterial or viral pneumonia), 'blocked nose' (sinusitis)

◆ **Skin problems**
Skin rashes, itching, anal itch/discomfort, Kaposi's sarcoma, folliculitis, seborrhoeic dermatitis, sepsis, warts, herpes infection, shingles

◆ **Swellings**
Swellings in the neck, groin, axilla (e.g. lymphadenopathy), parotid

◆ **Mouth / lips / gastro-intestinal problems**
Mouth sores, 'cold' sores, angular stomatitis, difficulty eating and swallowing (thrush), diarrhoea (gastro-enteritis), white and red patches (thrush)

◆ **Central nervous system problems**
Headache, blackouts, fits, faints, neck stiffness (e.g. meningitis, HIV brain infections, toxoplasmosis)

◆ **Mood changes**
Depression, memory loss, dementia

◆ **Pins and needles / shooting pains / numbness**
Peripheral neuropathy (e.g. HIV, Herpes zoster, drug side effects)

◆ **Visual disturbances**
Poor visual acuity, patchy vision (e.g. CMV, toxoplasmosis, retinitis)

◆ **Psychological disturbances**
Anxiety, depression, sleep problems, anger

◆ **Sexual problems**
Psychological disturbance, personal relationship problems, genital sores, discharges or itching (e.g. thrush, STIs)

◆ **Lack of energy**
Weakness, tiredness, lethargy (HIV infection), diarrhoea

These conditions are discussed in more detail in Chapter 7.

PRIMARY CARE FOR EARLY HIV

◆ Check and record the body weight

If there is weight loss think of the following:

◆ It may be a sign of an opportunistic infection, such as tuberculosis, PCP, chronic diarrhoeal disease or an underlying cancer.

◆ It may also be a sign of an increase in the activity of the HIV virus and a deterioration in the immune status and progression of the HIV disease.

◆ It may be associated with a loss of appetite, which may be due to a general deterioration.

◆ *There may be other causes as discussed on page 155.*

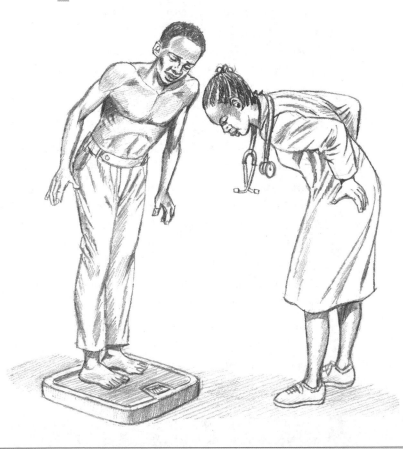

A stable body weight is an encouraging sign.
An unexplained and ongoing weight loss usually indicates a deteriorating condition with a poor prognosis. This must always be taken seriously.

◆ Examine specific areas thoroughly

The skin

HIV infection commonly causes skin problems. Some of these problems may occur early in the stage of HIV infection (before there is any significant immune-deficiency).

◆ **Skin problems may include conditions such as:**
- Seborrhoeic dermatitis
- Folliculitis, pustules, impetigo
- Fungal infections
- Parasitic infections (e.g. scabies)
- Viral infections (e.g. Herpes zoster and simplex, warts, molluscum contagiosum)
- Eczema and psoriasis
- The HIV-associated skin cancer (Kaposi's sarcoma)
- Drug reactions

Skin problems are discussed in more detail in Chapter 7.

Herpes zoster

Examination

It is important to thoroughly check the skin and include areas such as:

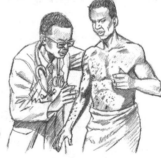

- The hairline and eyelid area (seborrhoeic dermatitis)
- The neck (pustules)
- The axilla and groin (fungal infection)
- The ano-genital area (warts, herpes)
- The chest and axilla (seborrhoeic dermatitis)
- The nails (fungal infection, paronychia)

Herpes zoster (shingles)

This is one of the common signs of immune-deficiency in patients with HIV.
The appearance of shingles almost always corresponds to a decreased CD4 count.

Kaposi's sarcoma

This often starts as dark bluish-black skin patches, usually ½ – 1 cm in size or longer.

Bruising or petechiae

These may be an indication of a low platelet count which may occur in the later stages of HIV infection.

Rashes and itchy skin conditions

These are common and are usually due to dry skin, folliculitis, seborrhoeic dermatitis, drug allergies, eczema and fungal infections (tinea).

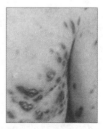

Kaposi's sarcoma

The mouth and teeth

The mouth is also a common area for early problems.

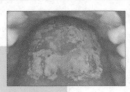

Oral thrush

◆ **Common mouth conditions include:**

   – *Candida albicans* (thrush)

   – Ulcers (aphthous)

   – Hairy leukoplakia

   – Kaposi's sarcoma (dark bluish-black
     swellings or patches may also occur
     on the palate and gums)

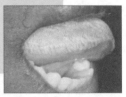

Hairy leukoplakia

Candida (thrush) in the mouth is a common sign of immune-deficiency, and does not usually occur unless the CD4 (T4) count is decreased (usually < 350 cells / mm³).

Examination

Check the mouth, lips and tongue

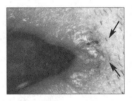

Angular stomatitis

◆ Check the corners of the mouth for
signs of malnutrition, infection (cracks, sepsis) and
fungal infection.

◆ Look for signs of herpes infection on the lips.

◆ Carefully examine the gums, palate, tongue,
tonsils and pharynx for thrush.

Check the condition of the teeth and gums (gingivitis)

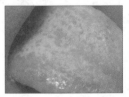

Oral thrush on tongue

◆ Any dental problem should be treated as early as
possible. This can help prevent problems and
secondary infection.

◆ If possible the patient should see a dentist or
dental therapist.

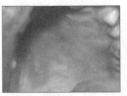

Palate thrush

**Remember the mouth is an important source of infection
and must be kept in a healthy state.**

The lymph nodes

◆ **Swollen and enlarged lymph nodes are important signs of HIV infection and of certain opportunistic infections and cancers. They could indicate:**

    – HIV infection itself (non-specific lymphadenopathy, usually non-tender)
    – Local skin infections (e.g. bacterial infection)
    – Upper respiratory tract infection
    – Tuberculosis
    – Secondary syphilis
    – Lymphoma
    There may be other causes, see page 146.

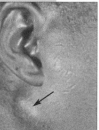

Lymphadenopathy

> **Shrinking of previously enlarged lymph nodes may also be a sign of progression of the HIV disease.**

Examination

Carefully examine the lymph nodes in the neck

◆ Below and behind the ears

◆ Under the jaw

◆ In the anterior (front) neck area

◆ In the posterior (back) neck area

◆ Above the clavicle

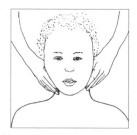

Examining lymph nodes in the neck

Also examine lymph nodes in the axilla, groin and above the elbow

◆ Lymphadenopathy is common and is usually due to the HIV disease. However, you need to be aware of other causes of lymphadenopathy and the conditions *(see page 146)*. Remember to consider tuberculosis if the glands are enlarged and/or matted in the neck.

◆ Lymphadenopathy which is non-tender, symmetrical (both sides), without any other abnormalities, is usually due to HIV alone.

◆ Parotid gland enlargement is also a feature of HIV infection.

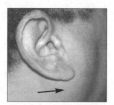

Parotid gland hypertrophy

There may be opportunistic infections or cancer (e.g. lymphoma) if the following are also present:

◆ Weight loss (TB, lymphoma)

◆ Night sweats and fevers (TB)

◆ Recurrent throat and mouth infections

◆ Tender, inflamed or rapidly changing nodes (acute infections)

◆ Enlarged liver or spleen (lymphoma)

◆ Grossly or asymmetrically enlarged or matted nodes (TB)

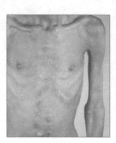

Wasting

The eyes

Examination

Check the eyelids to indicate conditions such as:

◆ Seborrhoeic dermatitis

◆ The development of a Kaposi's sarcoma

Check the retina

◆ Retinal signs are usually associated with advanced stages of HIV infection.

◆ Cytomegalovirus infection of the retina is usually seen in very advanced stages of AIDS, and usually indicates a very low CD4 count (less than 100 cells / mm³). Retinal signs of cytomegalovirus infection include irregular narrowing of the blood vessels. Vascular occlusions (blockages) with bleeding and white retinal exudates ('blotches and patches') and infarctions may occur. This may cause blindness.

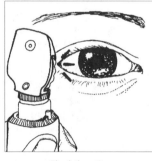

Check the retina

◆ Herpes zoster may affect the retina.

◆ Toxoplasmosis is another opportunistic infection which may affect the retina.

◆ HIV itself may also cause changes in the retina.

At times it may be difficult to fully examine the retina. If signs and symptoms suggest eye (retinal) disease, it is recommended to refer the patient to an ophthalmologist.

The genitals

It is important to examine the genital and peri-anal areas if indicated. Ulcerating sexually transmitted infections, such as syphilis, chancroid and herpes, are common infections in people who have HIV infection. Other STIs, such as gonorrhoea and non-gonococcal urethritis, are also commonly seen in people who have HIV.

Examination

Female genital area

◆ In women it is important to do an examination (speculum) of the vulva and vagina to look for candida infection. It is a common opportunistic infection of the genital tract.

◆ If a woman has candida infection in the mouth, then she may also have it in the vagina / vulva. Candida infection of the vulva / vagina is very common in advanced HIV disease and may present with a white curd-like discharge and / or pruritis vulvae (itching around the vulva).

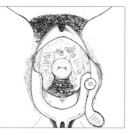

Candida

◆ Also look out for ulcers or signs of sexually transmitted infections (*see Chapter 12*). Genital herpes infection is also very common.

◆ Cancer of the cervix and infection with human papilloma virus (genital warts) are also important considerations in HIV-positive women. A PAP smear should be done every few years to detect signs of early cancer.

Male genital area

◆ Men may also occasionally present with candida infection which will appear on the glans of the penis (balanitis).

◆ Also look out for other STIs like chancroid (*see Chapter 12*).

◆ Herpes is also common in men.

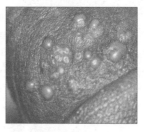

Penile herpes

Peri-anal area

◆ Remember also to examine the anal area for signs of sexually transmitted infections (ulcers, warts) or sepsis (abscess, fissure, fistula), especially if there are any symptoms of anal discomfort, pain, itching etc. Superficial peri-anal ulceration is common in advanced disease, and is usually due to viral infection, such as herpes and CMV.

PRIMARY CARE FOR EARLY HIV

The respiratory system

Respiratory infections are common which necessitates careful examination of the respiratory system.

> **Careful examination may alert you to respiratory disease such as:**
>
> ◆ Acute bacterial pneumonia (e.g. pneumococcal, *Haemophilus influenzae, atypical pneumonia*)
> ◆ Tuberculosis
> ◆ Viral pneumonia (e.g. cytomegalovirus)
> ◆ Parasitic infections, such as *Pneumocystis carinii*

Examination

◆ Observe the colour of the mucous membranes.

◆ Check the respiratory rate and movements.

◆ Percuss and auscultate the chest.

If other signs and symptoms, such as weight loss, fever and dyspnoea are present, a **chest X-ray** may be required. Many clinicians regard a chest X-ray as an important routine assessment in a newly diagnosed HIV-positive patient.

Note on tuberculosis:

Tuberculosis is a very common opportunistic infection in people with HIV infection. It may present in the usual way, but it **may also present in an unusual or atypical manner** e.g. acute onset, lower lobe pneumonia, sputum-negative or PPD negative skin test etc.
This is discussed in more detail in Chapter 11.

The abdomen

Examination

◆ A careful abdominal examination is important.

◆ Note the presence or absence of an enlarged liver or spleen. If either the liver or spleen is enlarged, this may be a sign of chronic infection or lymphoma.

◆ Neurological assessment

A brief and simple assessment may help to indicate any neurological involvement.

Test the following:

- Memory and the general mental state
- Pupil reaction
- Eye movement
- Visual acuity and field
- Sensation
- Signs of meningism
- Power and reflexes
- Gait (the way the person walks)

◆ General examination

You should also remember that HIV-infected people may also have many other conditions which are not especially associated with HIV.

A general body examination should also be done periodically to include:

- The cardio-vascular system, renal system and liver
- The extremities
- The nervous system
- The urine

◆ Investigations

It is useful to do some investigations to further assess the patient's condition, and to serve as a baseline for future comparison.

The investigations are carried out in order to:

- Assess various blood parameters – this may indicate important information or change as the disease progresses.
- Detect some silent or 'hidden' infection.
- Monitor the immune status of the body.
- Monitor the HIV status.

It is recognised that laboratory investigations are costly and may not always be affordable by the patient. Health care providers should be cost sensitive and avoid unnecessary tests or unnecessarily frequent investigations.

On the following page there is a list of the most common and important monitoring tests.

Monitoring the HIV and immune status, and other investigations

> **The following are the recommended routine investigations for assessing a patient with HIV:**
>
> *General*
>
> ◆ Full blood count (noting especially the lymphocyte and neutrophil count, haemoglobin level, and platelet count)
>
> ◆ Syphilis serology
>
> ◆ Liver enzymes (if ART is considered)
>
> *Immune function*
>
> ◆ Total lymphocyte count (if CD4 cell count is not available, *see page 77*)
>
> ◆ CD4 cell counts
>
> *HIV status*
>
> ◆ HIV RNA viral load (quantification)
>
> Other tests can be considered if indicated, such as a hepatitis B serology, PAP smear in women, a chest X-ray, a tuberculin skin test, renal and liver function.

As some of the tests listed above are not available or affordable in low resource health services, the following more readily available tests are recommended:

◆ A full blood count

A full blood count (FBC) is important as many conditions can be reflected in the FBC. The following are some of the most important HIV-related features:

Haemoglobin

The normal haemoglobin level is 12 – 18 g/dl.

The Hb level will indicate the presence of anaemia. HIV-infected people may also need to go onto medications (such as zidovudine, hydroxyurea, co-trimoxazole etc.) which can suppress or inhibit the bone marrow. It is therefore useful to know the usual haemoglobin level.

The marrow can also be suppressed by:

◆ HIV infection itself

◆ Tuberculosis, involving the bone marrow

◆ Other acute and chronic infections

White blood cell count

The normal white blood cell count (WCC) is 4 000 – 10 000 cells/mm³.

Changes in the white cell count may indicate bacterial, viral or parasitic infections.

The lymphocyte count is often reduced if there is immune-deficiency. A lymphocyte count below 1 200 cells/mm³ usually indicates immune-deficiency (CD4 < 200) in HIV infection *(see page 26)*.

Platelets

The normal platelet value is 140 000 – 440 000 cells/mm³.

A low platelet count, leading to thrombocytopaenia, is a common feature of advanced HIV.

◆ Tests for syphilis and other infections / conditions

A RPR/VDRL and other specific tests should be done to detect active syphilitic infection, which is a common association with HIV infection *(see Chapter 12)*. Abnormal neurological or psychological signs may occasionally be due to advanced syphilis (neuro-syphilis).

Syphilis, in the presence of HIV infection, may need more prolonged therapy *(see Chapter 12)*.

Some clinicians also do hepatitis B or C antigen and antibody serology. This is because hepatitis B is also often associated with HIV infection.

Liver and renal function can also be assessed, especially if ART is considered.

◆ CD4 (T4) cell count

The normal CD4 cell count ranges from 600 – 2 000 cells/mm³.

The CD4 cell count is one of the most valuable and useful markers of the state of the immunity in a patient with HIV/AIDS.

It is the best indicator of the risk for acquiring HIV-related opportunistic infections and other immune-deficiency disorders *(see pages 76 and 121)* as well as the best time to start ART. As the CD4 level drops, the risk for acquiring opportunistic infection increases. The onset of opportunistic infections is usually associated with CD4 counts below 350 – 400 cells/mm³. These are more common and more severe as the count drops further.

The table on page 121 illustrates the correlation between the CD4 cell count and the risk for specific diseases.

> **The CD4 cell count is an important indicator / predictor of the risk for acquiring opportunistic infections and when to start ART.**

The percentage of CD4 cells of the total lymphocyte count is also a useful measure. The percentage CD4 cells is normally more than 30% of the total lymphocyte count. Levels below 30% generally indicate immune-deficiency, and the lower the percentage, the more severe the deficiency.

The CD4 / CD8 ratio is another measure which may be considered. The normal ratio is greater than one, and ratios less than one indicate immune-deficiency.

The following must be considered when assessing the CD4 cell markers:

◆ The counts may vary and fluctuate. A single count is not often reliable of the actual state of immunity.

◆ Serial counts or trends over time are more reliable assessments of the immune status.

◆ The count may temporarily drop during pregnancy, infections, e.g. during active TB, and during other systemic conditions.

◆ The count usually drops progressively over time. The decline may be slow and steady, or it may be more rapid and acute. In some patients the count may show a transient rise or fall.

◆ A stable CD4 cell count is an encouraging sign. A progressively falling count usually indicates a more aggressive disease process.

◆ In some patients the count can rise or fall unpredictably.

◆ Unless the clinical condition is obvious, decisions on CD4 cell counts should involve at least 2 counts separated by 10 – 14 days.

There is more about the interpretation of CD4 cell counts on pages 77 – 78.

◆ HIV viral load

The HIV RNA viral load quantification is a relatively new test. This test measures the number of viral particles or 'copies' per mm^3 of blood. A rising viral load indicates very active HIV disease. High rising levels predict a more rapid development of immune-deficiency and a poorer outlook.

An individual **without** HIV infection will not have a detectable HIV viral load. Individuals **with** HIV may have levels which range:

– **from** undetectable levels (usually indicating a level too low for the test to detect, but not necessarily truly absent e.g. in a patient on ART. Current 'undetectable levels' are < 50 or < 400 copies / mm^3 (depending on laboratory).

– **to** very high levels such as 3 – 5 million copies / mm^3.

The diagram on page 76 shows the general pattern of CD4 cell counts and viral load over the time period of the disease.

The viral load is one of the most reliable indicators / predictors of the HIV progression. It predicts how rapidly the immune system will deteriorate. It is also helpful to assess efficacy and sensitivity of ART.

The viral load is very useful for:

◆ Assessing the severity of the HIV infection

    – a predictor for the development of immune-deficiency
      and disease progression

◆ The effect of ART and the ongoing monitoring of ART

◆ Detecting ARV drug resistance (*see pages 87 – 88*)

It should be noted that:

◆ The viral load can vary and fluctuate, and a single value should be
viewed with caution.

◆ There is a rise in viral load soon after HIV infection and it usually falls
soon thereafter.

◆ Even if the level is undetectable in the blood, (e.g. when on ART), it
does not mean the blood is free from HIV. The patient is still able to
spread the HIV.

◆ It does not detect HIV in other organ systems such as the lymph nodes,
liver, spleen, etc.

◆ The viral load should be monitored when necessary (e.g. for drug
therapy) at approximately 2 – 4 monthly intervals until stable and then
4 – 6 monthly. It should be done more frequently if clinically indicated.

◆ As new viral load assays become available, this test will become more
accurate and sensitive, and able to detect lower levels of virus. Current
viral load tests can detect the virus at levels as low as 50 copies / mm^3.
Some laboratories can only detect levels to 400 or less copies / mm^3.

◆ The blood for the test must be transported carefully to the laboratory.
It should be transported within 6 hours of taking the blood. Advice
should be obtained from the laboratory on the time delay and transport
of the specimen.

◆ The viral load test is not available in many outlying areas. It may be
unaffordable for some patients. Cheaper versions of viral load tests are
likely to be available in the future.

Relationship between viral load and CD4 cell count

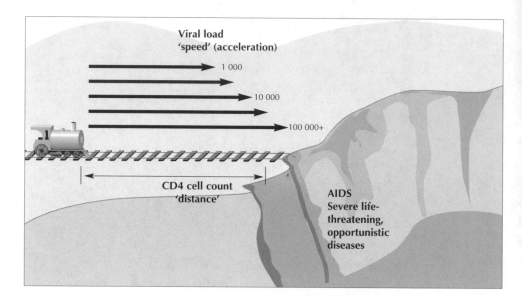

Pattern of patient 'wellness' relative to the phases of HIV infection, CD4 count and viral load

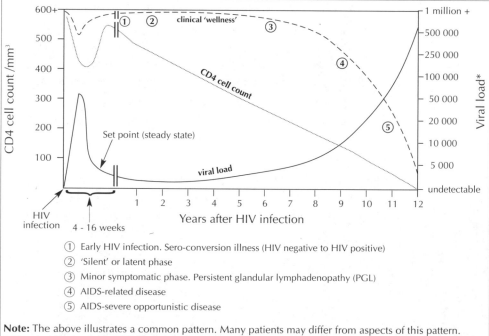

① Early HIV infection. Sero-conversion illness (HIV negative to HIV positive)

② 'Silent' or latent phase

③ Minor symptomatic phase. Persistent glandular lymphadenopathy (PGL)

④ AIDS-related disease

⑤ AIDS-severe opportunistic disease

Note: The above illustrates a common pattern. Many patients may differ from aspects of this pattern.
* The viral load values differ considerably in different patients.

◆ Chest X-ray

Respiratory disease may begin slowly without obvious signs or symptoms. A chest X-ray could be part of the initial assessment and is useful if there are other signs and symptoms suggestive of respiratory disease, such as weight loss, fever, dyspnoea, night sweats, cough.

It may help diagnose conditions such as:

◆ Acute bacterial or viral or fungal pneumonias

◆ Tuberculosis

◆ *Pneumocystis carinii* (PCP)

◆ Occasionally it may show up a hilar lymphadenopathy

◆ Provide a baseline for future comparison

Important investigations and their interpretation for the primary care of people with HIV infection		
Test	**Normal value**	**Interpretation**
FBC/Hb	12 – 18 g/dl	◆ Low if there is: – chronic infection – invasion of the marrow e.g. TB, cancer, HIV infection – bone marrow suppression
Lymphocytes	More than 1 500 cells/mm³	◆ Less than 1 200 often correlates with a low CD4 count (< 200) and may indicate: – immune-deficiency – the likelihood of opportunistic infection
Neutrophils	± 2 500 – 7 000 cells/mm³	◆ Raised in bacterial infection
Platelets	140 000 – 440 000 cells/mm³	◆ Low if there is: – advanced HIV disease – bone marrow infection – cancer (lymphoma)
CD4 (T4) cells	600 – 1 500 cells/mm³ or more	The CD4 cell count is the best indicator / predictor for the risk of developing opportunistic disease / infection, and the likely severity of such infections. ◆ 500 – 600 cells/mm³ – mild immune-deficiency – unlikely development of opportunistic infection

(continued on next page.)

Test	Normal value	Interpretation
CD4 (T4) cells (continued)	600 – 1500 cells / mm³ or more	◆ 300 – 500 cells/mm³ 　– moderate immune-deficiency 　– may expect some opportunistic infections, such as TB, candida (oral, vaginal), herpes, folliculitis ◆ 100 – 300 cells/mm³ 　– advanced or more severe immune-deficiency 　– expect opportunistic infection and some cancers (*see Chapter 7*) ◆ 0 – 100 cells/mm³ 　– very severe immune-deficiency 　– expect severe and frequent opportunistic infection e.g. cytomegaloviral disease, atypical mycobacterium, oesophageal candidiasis, etc.
HIV RNA viral load	No particles / copies detected (undetectable) (In HIV-positive patients the **trend** of viral load over time is also useful)	Absent HIV viral load indicates that there are too few particles to detect the virus. The viral load predicts the likelihood of disease progression and the development of immune-deficiency. ◆ 1 000 – 5 000 copies /mm³ 　– usually indicates low viral activity ◆ 5 000 – 15 000 copies /mm³ 　– moderate viral load and moderate activity ◆ 15 000 – 50 000 copies /mm³ 　– higher viral load and activity ◆ 50 000 – ± 1 million copies/mm³ or more 　– very high viral activity
RPR/VDRL	Negative	◆ Positive result usually indicates active syphilitic infection requiring treatment. Occasionally false negative results may also occur. *See also Chapter 12.*
Serology for hepatitis B and C is also useful (if available or affordable).	Absent or low IgG titre	◆ Low titre may indicate past exposure and risk for reactivation. ◆ High titre may indicate new infection.

Managing medical problems

The diagnosis and management of the many possible HIV-related conditions is a very important feature in the care of patients with HIV/AIDS.

The specific diagnosis and treatment of some of the more common conditions are discussed in Chapter 7

In general, most conditions are treated as usual. However, some conditions, such as syphilis, chancroid (*see Chapter 12*), diarrhoea, skin rashes, candida etc., may not respond well to the usual therapy. Higher doses, longer treatments or alternative medications may be required.

Anti-retroviral therapy (ART)

The purpose of ART (highly active ART – HAART) is to achieve HIV viral suppression and reduce the level of HIV RNA to as low a level as possible, for as long as possible. This in turn will result in less immune damage and will reduce any continued decline in the health status of the patient. It is therefore effective in delaying the onset of AIDS. ART must maintain very low and ideally undetectable HIV viral levels (viral load).

In recent years there have been exciting developments and discoveries in ART. This therapy is still expensive and often unaffordable to most people with HIV. As new medication becomes available, existing ones are becoming cheaper and affordable to more people. Hopefully these drugs will be more widely affordable and available.

It is possible that HIV may develop resistance to ART or the drugs may cause unwanted side effects or toxicity. For these reasons some patients cannot tolerate or use the medication, or may have to change the drug regimen.

Role of ART in *asymptomatic* patients who are NOT severely immune-deficient

- ART can inhibit and suppress HIV activity and replication. This will help to prevent further immune damage and result in a recovery of the immune capacity.

- Maintaining adequate or improved immune-function will in turn prevent disease progression, and promote ongoing wellness and health.

Role of ART in *symptomatic* patients WITH immune-deficiency

- ART may prevent further decline and damage to the immune status.

- ART may help to
    - promote some recovery of immune-status
    - improve immune-function and capacity
    - prevent disease progression.

- ART may reduce the frequency and severity of serious opportunistic infections.

- This results in improvement in general health, weight gain and increased appetite.
- This will prevent the need for hospital admissions and other costly health care. It will therefore facilitate important cost savings.

◆ ART is a complex issue and needs careful consideration

- ART usually requires a very committed and well-informed patient.
- Some drug regimens may require 2 – 3 different tablets, each needing to be taken 2 – 3 times a day. Some of the drugs are best taken on an empty stomach, and some not.
- Some patients may experience unwanted side effects or toxicity of the drugs.
- Treatment is currently ongoing and life-long. Compliance and strict adherence to therapy is often difficult to achieve.
- Some patients may find it difficult to tolerate the drugs due to unpleasant effects (nausea, headache etc.). They may need family or other support for successful adherence.
- There is always a possibility of developing viral resistance to the drugs. This would require a change in the regimen. Poor compliance and adherence to therapy is a common cause of resistance. Sub-optimal viral suppression will almost always lead to drug resistance. Drug resistance will eventually set in.
- Drug resistance may develop across a number of drugs, usually within the same group / class e.g. resistance to AZT may also result in resistance to other nucleoside reverse transcriptase drugs.
- In order to reduce the likelihood of drug resistance, combination therapy is used. Mono-therapy (single-drug) and dual therapy (two-drug) is not recommended.
- Drug therapy must be monitored regularly. HIV viral load is a good indicator as to whether the ART is effective, and whether the viral suppression is being maintained.
- Improved CD4 cell count indicates effective ART.
- Some ART drugs interact with other medications which are used in managing people with HIV. This is especially important with TB drugs (rifampicin).
- ART is costly, and many patients cannot afford it, or may not be able to afford optimal drug regimens.
- Patients must be committed to long-term ongoing treatment and strict adherence to therapy. They should also understand that therapy does not prevent HIV from being transmitted to their sexual partners.

ART should be monitored by doing regular HIV viral load measurements and CD4 cell counts. Ensure that the viral load is reduced and maintained at the lowest level possible, and that the CD4 cell count increases or is maintained at stable levels.

◆ Categories of drugs used for ART

There are currently three main categories of ARV drugs. However, medical science is discovering new agents e.g. fusion (T20) and integrase inhibitors. This means that the number of categories will change in future, and the number of drugs in each category is also undergoing rapid change. You will need to read about the latest developments in the medical literature, internet and other sources of information.

The 3 drug categories are:

Nucleoside reverse transcriptase inhibitors (NRTIs)

◆ NRTIs were amongst the first drugs developed. They include:
- zidovudine (Retrovir) (AZT)
- didanosine (Videx) (ddl)
- zalcitabine (Hivid) (ddC)
- lamivudine (Epivir) (3TC)
- stavudine (Zerit) (d4T)
- abacavir (Ziagen)
- tenofovir (newly released – not widely available yet)

Non-nucleoside reverse transcriptase inhibitors (NNRTIs)

◆ NNRTIs also disturb the life cycle of HIV by interfering with the reverse transcriptase enzyme in the replication process of the virus. They include:
- nevirapine (Virimune)
- efavirenz (Stocrin)
- delaviridine (not widely available yet)

Protease inhibitors (PIs)

◆ Protease inhibitors have added a new and potent addition to the ART option. They interfere with the formation of viable daughter virions in the life cycle replication of the virus. The following are currently used:
- indinavir (Crixivan)
- saquinavir (Invirase)
- nelfinavir (Viracept)
- ritonavir (Norvir). Usually used in lower dose to 'boost' some PIs *(see page 86)*
- amprenavir (Preclir)
- lopinavir / ritonavir (Kaletra)
- atazanavir (newly released – not widely available yet)

The above drugs can effectively block the replication of HIV. It is however uncertain whether replication is ever totally suppressed. Data suggests that once the ART is discontinued, viral replication is usually resumed, and viral loads usually rapidly rise again.

In order to maintain the ongoing viral suppression as long as possible, combinations of ART are recommended rather than a single-drug approach.

◆ When to start ART

The time to start ART is variable, and each patient needs to be assessed individually. However, the following principles for commencing therapy are provided.

General principles

It is best to start ART:

- *before* there is severe or advanced immune-deficiency
- *before* the viral load has increased to very high levels
- *before* the general clinical condition has deteriorated
- *if there are any* signs of conditions associated with significant immune-deficiency, such as moderate to severe oral thrush, recurrent severe herpes infections or shingles, recurrent infections such as pneumonia and diarrhoea
- *if there are any* AIDS-defining / indicator diseases *(see pages 102, 104, 118)*
- *for 9 – 12 months during* the acute primary HIV infection period *(see page 28)*, if this can be identified. This usually occurs 2 – 6 months after the HIV infection, and is associated with:
  - a significantly raised HIV viral load
  - a reduced CD4 cell count
  - clinical features described on *page 28.*

Asymptomatic patients

ART should be started if:

- The CD4 cell count approaches 250 cells/mm^3 or less.
- There is a *very* high viral load with a progressive drop in the CD4 cell count (with serial measurement).
- There is a r*apid and progressive* decline in the CD4 cell count (even if it has not yet reached 250 cells / mm^3). Some patients may start treatment at a CD4 count of 350 if the CD4 count is declining rapidly (> 100 cells / year).

Note: To assess a rapid decline in CD4 cells, the counts should be done at 2 monthly intervals. Do not rely on a single measurement only.

Symptomatic patients

As a general rule, ART should be started if the patient develops any significant clinical signs or symptoms related to immune-deficiency.

ART is recommended if:

- There are clinical signs of significant opportunistic infections or AIDS-defining diseases such as moderate to severe oral thrush, recurrent herpes infections or shingles, unexplained weight loss, severe infections such as pneumonia, ongoing diarrhoea, meningitis, severe neurological conditions, uncontrolled skin disorders, Kaposi's sarcoma, etc. *(see lists on pages 102, 104 and 118).*
- There are certain conditions which **may** only respond to ART, such as severe parotid gland enlargement, progressive peripheral neuropathy, dementia, warts etc.
- The CD4 cell count is below 250 cells / mm^3 *(see following page).*

Patients with advanced HIV disease

In patients who have advanced HIV disease, compared with patients with less advanced disease, ART is still likely to have important benefits and may be reasonably effective. However in the presence of advanced disease:

◆ The drugs are more likely to have a higher failure rate.

◆ There is more likelihood of side effects and toxic effects.

◆ The patient is more likely to have drug intolerance.

◆ Drug resistance is more likely to develop.

Note: It is therefore best to start ART earlier.

Symptomatic patient	Treatment
Presence of HIV-related symptoms, current or previous HIV-associated disease*	Treatment recommended
Primary infection†	Treatment recommended for 9 – 12 months
Asymptomatic patient	**Treatment**
CD4 count less than 200 cells / mm³	Treatment recommended
CD4 count 200 – 350 cells / mm³	Monitor CD4 count and commence treatment if the CD4 annual decline is in excess of the expected 20 – 80 cells / year, or if the CD4 count approaches 200 cells / mm³
CD4 cell count greater than 350 / cells / mm³	Postpone treatment

These include AIDS-defining illnesses (except TB), unexplained weight loss > 10% of body weight, unexplained diarrhoea lasting > 1 month, oral candidiasis or oral hairy leukoplakia.
† HAART started early in primary infection leads to viral suppression. This appears to maintain HIV-specific immunity in a significant proportion of cases, who become slow progressors with a low viral load after discontinuing HAART. The duration of treatment is uncertain at the present time.

Source: 'Antiretroviral therapy in adults.' Southern African Journal of HIV Medicine, July 2002, page 26

> **ART is likely to be more effective and successfully maintained for longer if begun before the patient is severely immune-deficient (CD4 ≥ 250) and before the clinical condition has deteriorated significantly. Drug toxicity and drug intolerance are also less common in patients who are clinically well without severe immune damage and with lower viral loads.**

◆ ART recommendations

Always use a combination of ART drugs

◆ Viral resistance is a continual concern, and this possibility is reduced if combination therapy is used.

◆ Mono-therapy (1 drug) with the currently available drugs will almost always lead to rapid development of drug resistance and is never recommended for ongoing care.

◆ Dual-therapy (2 drugs) may also lead to drug resistance, although it is likely to be more delayed than mono-therapy.

◆ Triple-therapy is ideally recommended.

Which drug regimens to use

◆ There is no international agreement as to any one particular or standard drug regimen.

◆ The choice of ART drug regimen is influenced by, and dependent on, many factors such as:

– what is affordable
– clinical history e.g. if there is a strong history of hepatitis, peripheral neuropathy, pancreatitis, bone marrow suppression, renal calculli (stones) or psychiatric disturbance, then it is best to avoid the ARV drugs which may have these side effects
– the stage of the disease i.e. the more advanced the stage of the disease, the greater the need for more potent drug regimens
– consideration of longer-term future drug options if the intial regimen ultimately fails e.g. you may want to use a PI-sparing regimen, and avoid some of their side effects (they can be used as a second-line option)
– convenience in drug dosage i.e. some regimens may only require daily or 2 x daily drug dosing which is more convenient than 3 x daily
– previous history of ART i.e. which drugs have been used in the past
– the 'first shot at ART should be your best shot'.

The following general options are provided. In situations where resources are very limited, the cost of the medication, the safety of the drugs and the regimen simplicity will influence choice. The cost for the medication has come down significantly in recent years, and more options are now becoming possible in situations where resources are limited.

The following is recommended:

NRTI and NNRTI combinations are usually recommended for starting therapy *(see also table on page 85).*

◆ Start with 1 drug from Category I **plus** 1 drug from Category II **plus** 1 drug from Category III *(see table on following page).*

◆ There have been reports of increased toxicity (lactic acidosis) with d4T and ddI in combination. This combination should be avoided if possible.

◆ Avoid triple NRTI regimens if possible.

Note: In primary HIV infection these drugs are given for 9 –12 months only.

Anti-retroviral regimens for the previously untreated patient

CATEGORY I (NRTI)	CATEGORY II (NRTI)	CATEGORY III (NNRTI)	CATEGORY IV (PI)
◆ Stavudine (d4T) ◆ Zidovudine (AZT)	◆ Didanosine (ddI) ◆ Zalcitabine (ddC) ◆ Lamivudine (3TC) ◆ Abacavir (ABC)†	◆ Nevirapine (NVP) ◆ Efavirenz (EFV)*	◆ Nelfinavir (NFV) ◆ Indinavir (IDV) ◆ Ritonavir (RIV) ◆ Saquinavir (SQV) (soft gel formulation) ◆ Lopinavir / ritonavir combination (Kaletra)

Teratogenic – should be avoided in women of childbearing potential unless using adequate intramuscular progestogens and barrier contraceptives, and only where no other anti-retrovirals are available.

†*Generally used if viral load is < 50 000 copies / mm³*

Source: Adapted from 'Antiretroviral therapy in adults.' Southern African Journal of HIV Medicine, July 2002, page 28

> **The ARV drug dosage and toxicity are outlined in the table on page 92.**

Commonly used regimens include:

PI sparing

◆ AZT **plus** 3TC **plus** NVP **or** EFV

◆ 3TC **plus** d4T **plus** NVP **or** EFV

◆ AZT **plus** ddI **plus** NVP **or** EFV

◆ 3TC **plus** ddI **plus** NVP **or** EFV

PI containing

◆ One drug from Category I, one drug from Category II or III,

  plus one drug from Category IV e.g.

  – AZT **plus** 3TC **plus** IDV

  – d4T **plus** 3TC **plus** Kaletra

  – AZT **plus** 3TC **plus** NFV

◆ Other combinations are also possible e.g.

  – 3TC **plus** Kaletra **plus** EFV

  Consult an HIV-experienced clinician.

Note: If you need an NRTI sparing regimen (because of toxicity / side effects), you can use 1 NNRTI **plus** 2 PIs.

Most clinicians prefer to keep the protease inhibitor drugs (Category IV) for later use in patients who:

◆ Develop resistance to the above NRTI and NNRTI regimens.

◆ Fail to tolerate these drugs due to toxicities or side effects.

◆ Develop treatment failure with these regimens.

The cost of the regimen often dictates what is possible.

◆ Indications for changing therapy

Treatment should only be changed in the following situations:

◆ There is patient-intolerance despite adequate and appropriate intervention.

◆ There are significant side effects and / or toxicity.

◆ There is treatment failure *(see page 88)*.

◆ Options for changing therapy

◆ Therapy may need to be changed when drug resistance emerges (always exclude poor compliance as the reason for drug failure before changing the drug regimen).

◆ When virological failure occurs, at least 2 of the drugs in the patient's regimen should be changed if possible. The clinician may choose to be guided by genotypic or phenotypic resistance testing if available.

Changing NRTIs (Categories I and II)

Initial agent	Change to new agent
Zidovudine	stavudine**
Stavudine	zidovudine**
Didanosine	lamivudine or zalcitabine
Lamivudine	didanosine* or zalcitabine*
Zalcitabine	abacavir, stavudine or zidovudine or other as determined by resistance testing
Abacavir	determined by resistance testing

*May exhibit reduced activity due to cross-resistance with lamivudine (3TC)
**May exhibit cross-resistance

Changing NNRTIs (Category III)

◆ There is broad cross-resistance between the currently available NNRTIs. Resistance to one NNRTI often prevents the use of another, unless there is resistance test data to the contrary.

◆ Individuals who fail an NNRTI-containing regimen may be candidates for a protease-inhibitor containing regimen. Resistance to 1 agent of this class effectively results in cross-resistance to all members of drugs in this category (that are currently available).

◆ Sequential use of these drugs is not recommended.

Changing PIs (Category IV)

◆ A major reason for regimens that contain protease inhibitors failing is poor adherence (often due to intolerance). This needs to be considered carefully before deciding to introduce an alternative PI-containing regimen.

◆ Pharmacological boosting of protease blood levels can be achieved by combining amprenavir, saquinavir, lopinavir and indinavir with low doses of ritonavir. Experience with these combinations is limited and readers should ask for advice on dosages.

◆ Monitoring ART

ART should be monitored with HIV viral load, CD4 cell counts and other supportive laboratory tests to monitor toxicity. These tests should be done every 2 – 3 months until stable then every 4 – 6 months if resources permit.

Viral load

◆ Viral load needs to be maintained at the lowest level possible, preferably at 'undetectable' levels. This needs to be sustained and ongoing.

◆ A progressive rise in viral load after 2 successive independent HIV viral load tests indicates treatment failure. This needs to be investigated as it might be due to drug resistance, poor adherence to drug compliance, or poor absorption of drugs.

◆ Avoid checking viral levels in the presence of intercurrent infections or recent immunisations (within 1 month of a vaccination) which may have caused the viral level to rise.

CD4 cell counts

◆ A favourable CD4 cell count is the desired outcome of ART, and this should be monitored regularly. Ideally, the CD4 cell count should improve after ART has started, and be maintained at higher levels. This should be ongoing and sustained.

◆ A progressively falling CD4 cell count shown by at least 2 independent counts at least 2 weeks apart is evidence of treatment failure. It needs to be investigated as above.

◆ Avoid checking CD4 counts in the presence of intercurrent infections where the counts can drop during the infections.

Supportive laboratory tests

The following tests should be done if resources permit. The objective of these tests is to monitor drug toxicity. Such tests should be done every 4 – 6 months.

◆ Bone marrow toxicity
  – full blood count (anaemia, thrombocytopaemia, lymphocytopaenia)
◆ Liver toxicity and function
  – liver function tests (liver enzymes – transaminases, LDH, bilirubin)
◆ Renal toxicity and function
  – urea, creatinine and electrolytes
◆ Other tests if indicated (if symptoms or signs are present) to detect pancreatitis (serum amylase), lactic acidosis (lactate levels) etc.

The viral load should ideally drop at least a full log value (10 times the previous level) within the first 8 – 12 weeks after commencing therapy. Ideally viral load should drop to undetectable levels and be maintained at these levels. However this is not always possible. The CD4 cell count should be maintained at improved levels or at the very least have stopped declining. This level must be maintained and sustained.

◆ ART drug failure

◆ At the onset of therapy the viral load should reduce significantly. Ideally the load should reduce by at least 1 log (10 times) by approximately 8 – 12 weeks after the start of ART.

– if the viral load does not reduce significantly within the first 3 – 4 months of therapy, then this initial therapy should be considered to have failed.
– alternative regimens should then be considered.

◆ ART failure is shown by:

– a continual rise in viral load
– **and / or** a declining CD4 cell count in the presence of a high or increasing viral load.

◆ A deteriorating clinical condition is also suggestive of failed therapy. In such situations the following should be considered:

– the laboratory may be able to assist in testing for drug-resistant assays, and identifying the specific drug resistance in the patient. This will inform the clinician on which drugs to avoid.
– changing to another drug regimen which is significantly different to the one in current use, e.g. consider using one or more protease inhibitors, if they were not previously used; or consider a non-nucleoside RTI if not previously used; or consider a different combination of NRTIs *(see page 86)*.
– consult a specialist HIV clinician or specialised HIV care unit.
– always suspect inadequate adherence to taking the ART drugs.

◆ Side effects / toxicity of ART

Most of the ARV drugs are potentially toxic and may cause side effects. Most patients are able to tolerate the drugs well. The clinician and the patient must always be on the lookout for the development of side effects. There are often milder self-limiting side effects in the first 4 – 8 weeks after starting ART. ART side effects and toxicity usually disappear if the drugs are stopped.

Milder side effects and toxicities

These are likely to occur in the first few weeks after starting the ARV regimens and include:

◆ Indigestion, change in bowel movements, diarrhoea, nausea

◆ Skin rashes

◆ Headache and dizziness

◆ Weakness, tiredness, lethargy

More serious side effects or toxicities

These may include:

◆ Abdominal pain which is more likely to be in the central upper abdominal area (NRTIs);
  – also loss of appetite, nausea and vomiting, i.e. pancreatitis .

◆ Abnormal feeling in the hands and feet and possibly around the mouth (NRTIs);
  – loss of feeling, feelings of 'pins and needles' or feeling that the arm or foot has gone to sleep
  – shooting pains in the hands and feet, or pains on the soles and palms.

These problems may continue to get worse and rise up the foot towards the knee or up the arm towards the elbow, i.e. peripheral neuropathy.

◆ Nausea, vomiting and vague abdominal pain (NRTIs);
  – possibly starting to breathe more quickly and deeply, i.e. lactic acidosis.

◆ Skin rashes which may be very severe or may present with large red blisters i.e. Steven Johnson syndrome or other drug allergic rashes (nevirapine).

Other possible serious side effects / toxicities

These may include:

◆ Bone marrow depression (bleeding, anaemia) (AZT)

◆ Abnormal metabolic disorders resulting in the following disorders:
  – lipid and fat metabolism (NRTIs, PIs)
  – diabetes (PIs)
  – raised cholesterol and uric acid (PIs)
  – reduced bone density (PIs)

◆ Mitochondrial damage and malfunction that may cause the following:
  – peripheral neuropathy and dementia
  – macular complications and hypotonia
  – myopathy and cardiomyopathy
  – liver disease and lactic acidosis
  – pancreatitis, pancytopaenia and renal disease

These conditions are usually associated with NRTI ARV drugs.

◆ Renal calculi (indinavir)

◆ Hepatitis (nevirapine)

Interaction with other drugs

◆ ARV drugs may interact with other drugs causing reduction or elevation of blood levels and other pharmacological dynamics. Clinicians will need to become familiar with the pharmacology of ARV medications.

Lactic acidosis

◆ NRTI drugs may cause lactic acidosis which can be life threatening. It is more common in patients who are on AZT, ddI and d4T.

◆ Symptoms may include malaise, nausea and vomiting, abdominal pain and later signs of acidosis i.e. hyperventilation.

◆ There is usually a lactic acidaemia, raised lactate levels, raised LDH and elevated liver transaminase levels.

◆ If lactate levels rise above 5 mmol / l with symptoms, the NRTI should be discontinued. If greater than 10 mmol / l, it must definitely be stopped. Other causes of the symptoms should also be investigated.

Immune reconstitution syndrome

◆ This is a well-documented syndrome following the commencement of ART in patients with AIDS and other chronic intracellular infections such as TB, cryptococcus, CMV virus and hepatitis B and C.

◆ With reconstitution of the immune system, a 'boosted' immune response takes place in the tissue where these intracellular infections are based. It usually occurs between 2 – 11 months after the commencement of ART.

◆ Symptoms are related to an acute inflammatory response in the tissue as a result of the rejuvenated immune response and may include fever, wasting (cahexia), local lymphadenopathy, tissue damage and necrosis.

◆ In dormant CMV, reports of uveitis have occurred.

◆ Patients with hepatitis B and C have experienced tender hepatomegaly and raised transaminases.

◆ In TB it may paradoxically worsen the TB disease initially (increase TB infiltrates, lymph adenopathy increase etc.). A delay in the commencement of ART in TB patients may be required *(see page 255)*.

◆ Immune reconstitution syndrome is usually associated with improved CD4 count and lowering of viral load.

◆ Treatment with anti-inflammatory medication or steroids may be necessary. The prognosis is usually good and allows for the continuation of ART.

Note: In general, ART drug dosages and regimens will need to be adjusted if there is compromised liver or renal function. Expert assistance should be sought in these situations.

Potential side effects of ARVs

Side effect / complication	NRTI	NNRTI	PIs
Myelosuppression	Yes	No	No
GI intolerance	Yes	Yes	Yes
Pancreatitis	Yes	No	No
Peripheral neuropathy	Yes	No	No
Allergic reaction	Rare potential for hypersensitivity reaction with abacavir	Yes	Rare
Lipoatrophy	Yes	Unknown	Unknown
Lactic acidosis	Yes	No	No
Lipodystrophy	Yes	Unknown	Yes
Raised cholesterol and triglyceride	Unknown	Yes: efavirenz	Yes
Insulin resistance	No	No	Yes
Neuro-psychiatric manifestations	No	Yes: efavirenz	Yes

Also note the following about:

NRTIs

◆ Major potential side effects include pancreatitis, peripheral neuropathy and lactic acidosis (may present with malaise, nausea, hyperventilation) due to mitochondrial damage – *see above*)

NNRTIs

◆ **Nevirapine**
  – Hepatitis is a concern as it can be fatal.
  – Nevirapine should not be given if there is any liver dysfunction / disease.
  – Before using a nevirapine-containing regimen, the liver function (transaminase levels) need to be checked and the drug avoided if these levels are significantly raised.
  – Skin rashes – to avoid skin rash it is best to give 200 mg nevirapine for the first 2 weeks, and then increase to 400 mg.

◆ **Efavirenz**
  – Should be avoided if there is a history of any psychiatric illness (depression, sleep disorders)

PIs

◆ Metabolic disturbances outlined in the *table above* are major considerations. Indinavir may also cause renal calculi so patients should drink large amounts of water (2 litres / day) and the drug avoided when dehydration is possible, e.g. underground mining.

Doses and toxicities of commonly available ARVs

ART	Drug	Dose	Toxicity
Nucleoside Reverse Analogue Transcriptase Inhibitors (RTIs)	abacavir (Ziagen)	300 mg 12 hourly	Hypersensitivity – fever, rash, GIT; hypotension; lipodistrophy
	zidovudine (AZT, ZDV, Retrovir)	250 – 300 mg 2 x daily (in combination with lamivudine)	Anaemia, neutropaenia, nausea, vomiting, fatigue, peripheral neuropathy (bone marrow suppression)
	didanosine (ddI, Videx)	200 mg 2 x daily OR 400 mg daily (take on an empty stomach)	GI disturbances, pancreatitis, peripheral neuropathy, nausea, diarrhoea, lactic acidosis
	zalcitabine (ddC, Hivid)	0,75 mg 3 x daily	Rash, oral ulcers (stomatitis), peripheral neuropathy
	stavudine (d4T, Zerit)	40 mg 2 x daily	Peripheral neuropathy, lactic acidosis
	lamivudine (3TC, Epivir)	150 mg 2 x daily (or in combination with zidovudine)	Minimal
Non-nucleoside Reverse Transcriptase Inhibitors (NNRTIs)	nevirapine (Viramune)	200 mg daily for 14 days, then 200 mg 2 x daily	Skin rash, hepatitis, Steven Johnsons Syndrome
	efavirenz (Stocrin)	600 mg nocte	CNS effects, dizziness, transient rash, Teratogenic
Protease Inhibitors (PIs)	saquinavir (Invirase)	600 mg 2 – 3 x daily	None or minimal, GI distrubances, headache
	nelfinavir (Viracept)	750 mg 8 hourly with meals	Diarrhoea
	indinavir* (Crixivan)	800 mg 3 x daily on an empty stomach	Renal stones, GI disturbances, increased bilirubin, lipodystrophy
	ritonavir* (Norvir)	400 – 600 mg 2 x daily with food 100 mg as a 'booster'	Perioral prasthesiae, nausea, headache, lipodystrophy, CPK increase
	lopinavir / ritonavir (Kaletra)	400 mg / 100 mg 2 x daily with food	long-term metabolic side effects

Note: Some of the dosages may change when used in combination.

* NB: Indinavir, ritonavir and other PIs interact with a large number of drugs. They need to be used with caution. Read the package insert carefully before prescribing for your patient.

◆ ARV drug interaction with other commonly used drugs

Many of the ARV drugs may react with other commonly used medication. Clinicians should consult the drug information inserts. Some of the protease inhibitors may cross-react with many different drugs.

See page 255 for TB drug reactions.

See pages 230 – 232 for using ART in pregnancy.

> **ART is all about risk management.**
> **It is important that there is a balance between the risks of the**
> **disease and the risks and considerations of ART (optimal time to**
> **start therapy, drug regimen, cost, side effects, etc.).**

Preventing opportunistic infections

Even if patients are generally asymptomatic, they could still have an advanced stage of immune-deficiency. They may also have some 'silent' opportunistic infections, e.g. oral thrush. They may have had some infections (e.g. shingles) which have cleared up on their own.

A low CD4 (T4) count (< 200) or a low lymphocyte count (< 1 200) is indicative of immune-deficiency. In the absence of these tests, conditions such as oral thrush, seborrhoeic dermatitis, herpes simplex (cold sore) or Herpes zoster (shingles), may alert you to immune-deficiency.

People with HIV infection and advanced stages of immune-deficiency (CD4 cell count less than 200 cells/mm³) can be offered prophylaxis for conditions such as thrush (if present), pneumocystis and toxoplasmosis. Prophylaxis of 'TB' is usually started earlier. Many clinicians recommend TB prophylaxis at any time or when the CD4 count drops below 400 cells / mm³.

It is also possible to offer patients immunisation against various diseases such as influenza.

Prophylaxis of opportunistic infection is discussed in more detail in Chapter 6.

The graph indicating prophylaxis of opportunistic infections relative to the CD4 cell count and onset of signs is on the following page.

Prophylaxis for opportunistic infections relative to the CD4 cell count and / or the likely onset of common or important signs / diseases.

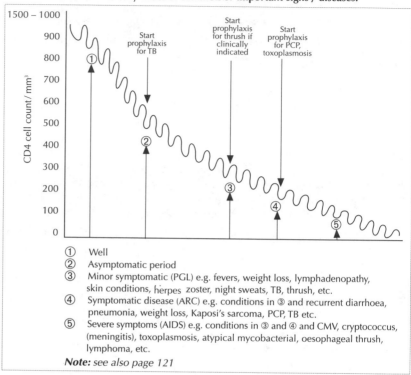

① Well
② Asymptomatic period
③ Minor symptomatic (PGL) e.g. fevers, weight loss, lymphadenopathy, skin conditions, herpes zoster, night sweats, TB, thrush, etc.
④ Symptomatic disease (ARC) e.g. conditions in ③ and recurrent diarrhoea, pneumonia, weight loss, Kaposi's sarcoma, PCP, TB etc.
⑤ Severe symptoms (AIDS) e.g. conditions in ③ and ④ and CMV, cryptococcus, (meningitis), toxoplasmosis, atypical mycobacterial, oesophageal thrush, lymphoma, etc.

Note: see also page 121

Advice on self care, safer sexual practices and a 'wellness' programme

◆ Self care – a 'wellness' programme

It is important to continually advise patients about how they can support and help their bodies to remain well as long as possible. This means that they should try to live healthy lifestyles and prevent re-infection with HIV.

Advise patients about the following:

Have a healthy diet

◆ If possible patients should try and eat healthy foods.

◆ They should eat plenty of fresh foods with lots of fruit and vegetables, and maintain a balanced diet.

Consider nutritional supplements

◆ The use of multivitamin supplements and 'immune boosting' medication has doubtful value.
They are however useful if the patient does not have a good balanced diet.

- Some patients feel better taking these supplements and for this reason they are listed.
- Vitamin A supplementation may have some benefit in reducing mother to child transmission, however this is as yet still uncertain.

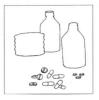

- Antioxidants, Sutherlandia plant extracts and selenium supplements etc. are used by some patients, but there is no real evidence that they have any significant impact on the disease progress.

Avoid smoking

- Tobacco smoke harms the lung's immunity.
- Respiratory infections account for a large proportion of opportunistic infections. A healthy respiratory system is important.
- Patients should try to stop smoking or reduce the number of cigarettes per day.

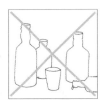

Avoid alcohol intoxication

- Too much alcohol is harmful.
- Many drugs used in HIV disease are possibly harmful to the liver. It is important to keep the liver as healthy as possible.
- Advise patients to avoid alcohol intoxication.

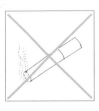

Keep fit and well exercised

- Exercise and fitness help to keep the body in good shape and will help patients to feel well and strong.
- However, advise patients not to over-stress the body, especially with symptoms of disease, such as diarrhoea, cough, fever etc.

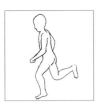

Avoid taking unnecessary drugs

- Drugs can be harmful and may have side effects.
- Patients should only take medicines which are advised by the health worker.

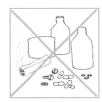

Have lots of rest and sleep

- Rest regularly and get enough sleep.
- If at all possible patients should avoid too much stress.

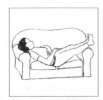

Have a positive mental attitude

◆ A positive mental attitude promotes health and wellbeing, and helps to keep patients well for longer.

Alternative therapies

◆ Alternative therapy such as acupuncture, massage, homeopathy, aluverdic medicine and traditional healing etc. may be useful, but have as yet unproven value for HIV/AIDS care.

◆ They could be considered as supportive therapy and should not be discouraged in patients with strong beliefs in such therapy.

◆ Time and research will help to understand the contribution of these therapies. Research has been carried out on the following:

– The African Potato (Hypoxis) claimed to boost the immune system. But the efficacy and safety study of Hypoxis was stopped at eight weeks as a result of the development of serious bone-marrow suppression in the majority of patients.

– Garlic powder thought to have antiviral properties, was shown to damage gastric mucosa. Garlic supplements, given for over 2 months, may lengthen bleeding time and interact with ARVs.

– Onions and olive oil also failed to show immune boosting properties. Large doses of onions may cause chronic diarrhoea and intestinal distension. Taken together they are likely to be harmful, and may in fact hasten the onset of full-blown AIDS.

Seek early treatment for medical problems

◆ It is important to seek treatment for medical problems as soon as possible.

◆ Many of the conditions are effectively treated if they are diagnosed early enough.

◆ Encourage patients to come for treatment as soon as they notice any problems.

◆ Safer sexual practices

It is important for patients to prevent spreading the HIV infection to others.
It is also harmful to get repeated HIV infection from others.

Give advice about the following:

Protection

◆ If the patient is having vaginal or anal sex, he / she must protect himself / herself and the partner by using a condom.

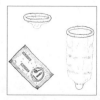

Alternative sexual methods

◆ Try to have enjoyable sex and sexual pleasure without penetration.
This can be achieved through masturbation and body sex (thigh sex).

◆ It is also safe to be caressed and to caress one's partner.

◆ If a man wants oral sex it is safest if he uses a condom.

Anal sex

◆ Try to avoid having anal sex if possible, or use double-strength condoms.

Alcohol and dagga (ganja, zoll or marijuana)

◆ These should be discouraged as they can influence people to have unsafe sex.

Support, counselling and referral

◆ Support and counselling should be part of each visit

Try to offer patients as much support as possible. Let them know that you or your co-workers will be available for them whenever they need advice, support and care.

Many people with HIV have fears, anxieties, worries and other problems. They need to be kept adequately informed about their condition, and they must be encouraged to be part of the treatment and management decisions.

It is common for patients in the asymptomatic phase to neglect follow-up checks and monitoring. Occasionally patients 'disappear' and are not seen again. Support and counselling can help to encourage patients to maintain regular contact and medical monitoring.

A patient may have problems with his / her sex life or with family or friends. Advice may be needed on how to cope with work and the employer. Sleep may also become a problem.

Encourage the patient to share his / her feelings and problems. If you are unable to deal with them, there may be others, or other services or organisations, who could provide the necessary support or advice *(see the following page)*.

◆ Counselling family members

Remember, a patient's husband, wife or lover, family members or friends may also need support, advice or counselling.

ART adherence is usually most effective if there is family support for the patient on ART.

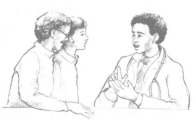

◆ Other agencies or organisations

People with HIV may need the following:
- legal assistance (e.g. to draw up a will)
- social welfare advice (e.g. for pensions or disability)
- advice and support for other medical and social problems

There are many other agencies and organisations who offer HIV-positive people counselling, advice and support (*see page 116*). These organisations should be sought out and used.

Counselling is discussed in more detail in Chapter 13.

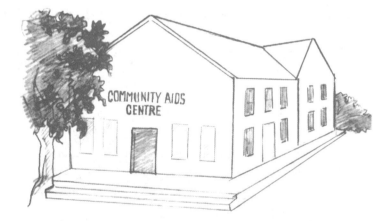

HIV-positive people may remain well and asymptomatic for a long time. Most of these people in the absence of ART will eventually start developing signs and symptoms of immune-deficiency. This may take between 3 and 8 years (even up to 10 years), from the time of the first HIV infection.

The clinical care of people with more advanced or symptomatic HIV/AIDS is discussed in the next chapter.

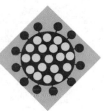

Chapter 6

PRIMARY CARE FOR ADVANCED (SYMPTOMATIC) HIV DISEASE AND AIDS

Principles of management

Regular medical checks

Assessing the immune status and stage of HIV disease

Assessing the HIV viral load

Anti-retroviral therapy (ART)

Preventing opportunistic infections

Treating opportunistic infections and other
HIV-related conditions

Support, counselling and referral

Home-care, day-care, hospital or hospice

World Health Organisation Staging System
for HIV Infection and Disease

The Center for Disease Control (USA)
case definition of AIDS

Correlation of HIV-related diseases / conditions with
CD4 cell counts

Principles of management

Patients can have a very varied clinical course. Some patients may develop a predicted course with a slow and steady decline; others may remain very well for a long time and then decline very rapidly. A proportion of patients are 'slow progressors' and remain well and healthy for many years.

Also some patients may have a severe life-threatening condition, and recover and remain in reasonable health for a long period of time.

HIV/AIDS is an unpredictable condition and the unexpected can occur. There are very few 'rules' with this disease.

It is not easy to determine what course each patient will follow, but some of the laboratory tests and the clinical picture described in *Chapter 5* will assist in making this assessment.

Regular medical checks

◆ General assessment

- ◆ The patient should be reviewed regularly depending on the clinical state.
- ◆ Well individuals can be seen at 3 – 4 monthly intervals.
- ◆ Patients who are on active therapy (e.g. ART, prophylaxis) or are symptomatic of opportunistic infections will need more regular follow-up at times. This may be necessary every 4 – 8 weeks or more often if not clinically well.

Physical examination

At each visit you must repeat a general physical examination. This examination was discussed in detail in *Chapter 5*.

- ◆ You will need to give particular attention to the weight, skin, mouth, lymph node enlargement, retinal changes and signs of respiratory infection.
- ◆ You will need to do an abdominal and a genital examination (if there are symptoms of genital disease).
- ◆ It is also important to do periodic neurological assessments.

Laboratory tests

Various laboratory tests will be necessary. The clinical condition of the patient will usually determine what needs to be done.

- ◆ Some tests may be needed to monitor the disease process such as CD4 cell count and HIV viral load.
- ◆ Other tests are to monitor for side effects of some drugs or for the general state of health e.g. a full blood count, and sometimes a renal function, liver function etc.
- ◆ Some tests may be needed to diagnose clinical conditions such as sputum microscopy, blood cultures, lumbar puncture, chest X-ray etc.

◆ Looking for signs and symptoms of HIV-associated conditions

At each visit, carefully enquire and examine for signs and symptoms of the common conditions associated with HIV-related disease *(see diagram on page 103, and the lists below and on page 104).*

Assessing the immune status and stage of HIV disease

The CD4 cell count is a very valuable and useful indicator of immune-capacity in people with HIV. It is the most reliable predictor for the risk of developing opportunistic infections and symptomatic disease. This has been discussed in more detail in *Chapters 3 and 5*. Various clinical management decisions, such as commencing prophylaxis (prevention) therapy or ART, may be considered if the CD4 counts are known.

Unfortunately CD4 cell counts are costly and need sophisticated laboratory technology. In many health services, especially in rural and low socio-economic areas, CD4 cell counts may not be available or affordable. In these situations you will need to be guided by:

- the lymphocyte count (see below)
- the patient's clinical condition
- looking out for signs and symptoms of opportunistic infections (which develop if there is immune-deficiency).

The following conditions are VERY SUGGESTIVE OF IMMUNE-DEFICIENCY and advanced HIV disease in an HIV-positive adult:

- Recurrent or persistent *Candida albicans* (thrush) in the mouth and vagina
- Hairy leukoplakia (white plaques) on the tongue *(see page 137)*
- Herpes zoster (shingles) and herpes simplex (cold sores)
- Skin rashes e.g. itchy (pruritic) maculo-papular rashes, seborrhoeic dermatitis, fungal infections (tinea), warts, molluscum contagiosum
- Weight loss for no obvious reason (usually more than 10% of body weight)
- Fever or night sweats
- Diarrhoea (ongoing for many days or weeks)
- Dyspnoea, tachypnoea and cough (ongoing for more than a month)
- Peri-anal conditions e.g. abscess, fistula and fissure
- Pulmonary and extra-pulmonary tuberculosis
- Genital ulcers which do not heal with treatment
- Neurological problems, such as memory loss, personality changes, severe weakness, fits and peripheral neuropathy
- Anaemia (pallor) for no obvious reason

Most of these conditions are usually associated with a low lymphocyte count (less than 1 200 cells/mm³) and a low CD4 (T4) cell count (less than 200 cells/mm³).

Conditions commonly suggestive of immune-deficiency and advanced HIV disease

Eye conditions

Retinitis

Mouth conditions

Herpes simplex (cold sore)
Candida albicans (thrush)
Ulcers (aphthous)
Leukoplakia (tongue)
Gum infections
Parotid gland enlargement

Oesophagus

Dysphagia
Oesophagitis (due to herpes /
candidia and other infections

Respiratory conditions

Pneumonia, especially
pneumococcal infection
Pneumocystis carinii
Tuberculosis

Enlarged spleen / liver

Lymphoma

Gastro-intestinal conditions

Diarrhoea (more than 4 weeks)
Pain – oesophagitis; mycobacterial
infection (MAC, TB) etc.

Muscle problems

Wasting of muscles

General problems

Weight loss (greater than 10%
body weight)
Persistent unexplained fever and
night sweats

Central neurological conditions

Memory loss
Personality changes
Severe weakness
Fits
Meningitis

Lymphadenopathy

Skin conditions

Seborrhoeic dermatitis
Folliculitis
Itchy (pruritic) maculo-
papular rashes
Dermatitis (eczema)
Fungal infections (tinea)
Warts
Herpes zoster (shingles)
Kaposi's sarcoma

Genital / anal problems

Candida albicans (thrush)
Genital ulcers
Peri-anal conditions e.g.
abscess
fistula
fissure
herpes
CMV

Peripheral neuropathy

Hands
Feet

Common early clinical signs of immune-deficiency include the presence of recurrent or persistent oral candida (thrush), herpes infection (cold sores) and Herpes zoster (shingles). These conditions usually correlate well with a low CD4 cell count (less than 300 cells/mm³) in people with HIV infection.

> **Candida (thrush) in the mouth is usually one of the first signs of advanced immune-deficiency.**

The following conditions are AIDS-DEFINING. THEY ARE DIAGNOSTIC OF AIDS AND DEFINITELY INDICATE severe IMMUNE-DEFICIENCY in an HIV-positive adult:

◆ Kaposi's sarcoma (skin, palate, lungs, GIT)

◆ *Pneumocystis carinii* pneumonia

◆ Recurrent bacterial pneumonia (pneumococcal pneumonia is common)

◆ Candida infection in the oesophagus

◆ Herpes simplex with muco-cutaneous ulcer for > 1 month

◆ Retinitis due to cytomegalovirus, herpes, HIV

◆ Chronic diarrhoeal disease

◆ Meningitis/encephalitis due to cryptococcal or toxoplasmosis infection

◆ Pulmonary, miliary or extra-pulmonary tuberculosis

◆ Dementia for no other reason (HIV encephalopathy)

◆ Wasting

◆ Some other cancers, such as lymphoma, are also associated with AIDS. These may present with enlarged lymph nodes, liver and/or spleen.

◆ Toxoplasmosis

See also AIDS-defining conditions in the WHO Staging System for HIV Infection and Disease *(page 118)* and the Center for Disease Control case definition *(pages 119 – 120)*.

The above conditions are the most common and are closely associated with advanced HIV infection and AIDS. However, you may also find other less common or unusual findings.

These conditions above are usually associated with a low lymphocyte count (less than 1 000 cells/mm³) and a very low CD4 (T4) cell count (less than 200 cells/mm³ and often below 100 cells / mm³).

The illustration on page 103 and the table on page 121 provide a correlation between the CD4 cell count and HIV-related diseases and conditions.

◆ Diagnosing the AIDS phase / stage

The patient has developed AIDS if the following are present:

- ◆ The patient is HIV positive
- ◆ The CD4 count is 200 cells/mm³ or less

  and/or

- ◆ There is an AIDS-defining disease (*see page 118*).

The Center for Disease Control (USA) Case Definition of AIDS can be found on pages 119 – 120.

Assessing the HIV viral load

The use and value of the HIV viral load has been discussed in detail on page 74.

◆ Other laboratory investigations

Besides the CD4 cell count and HIV viral load, other laboratory tests are done in order to:

- ◆ Monitor body function
- ◆ Investigate any abnormal clinical findings

Tests to monitor body function

Some laboratory tests are useful in assessing normal body function. These can be done periodically if there is a need:

- ◆ **A full blood count**
  e.g. To check for anaemia, thrombocytopaenia and signs of marrow depression (especially if using drugs such as AZT).

- ◆ **Urea and electrolytes**
  e.g. To check kidney function or electrolyte level if there is diarrhoeal disease.

- ◆ **Liver function**
  e.g. If the patient is on various medications which may be affected by liver disease, such as ketoconazole (Nizoral), nevirapine etc.

- ◆ **Serum albumin**
  This may be low in advanced stages of HIV disease, especially if there is unexplained oedema.

- ◆ **Other tests**
  Laboratory tests such as serum amylase, lactose dehydrogenase (LDH), muscle enzymes, lactate levels etc., may also be assessed if clinically indicated.

PRIMARY CARE FOR LATE HIV/AIDS

Tests to investigate any abnormal clinical findings

Laboratory tests to assist in the diagnosis of various clinical conditions may be required e.g.

- **Blood cultures**
- **Urine**
  For microscopy cells and culture
- **Stools**
  For microscopy cells and culture
- **CSF (lumbar puncture)**
  For microscopy, cells, glucose, electrolytes, protein and culture.
  For RPR/VDRL (if syphilis is suspected).
  For cryptococcal antigen and India ink stain (cryptococcal) if indicated.
- **Sputum**
  For cells and acid fast bacilli, fungal studies and culture
- **Radiological investigations**
  Such as chest X-rays and scans
- **Biopsy**
  Of the skin, bone marrow or lymph nodes if necessary
- **Bronchial washings (PCP diagnosis)**

Remember many of these tests and investigations are expensive and may not be available in many areas. You may have to rely on your clinical judgement.

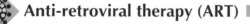

Anti-retroviral therapy (ART)

Anti-retroviral therapy (ART) should be offered if possible.
This has been outlined in Chapter 5.

Preventing opportunistic infections

Another important feature of the care of people in advanced stages of HIV infection is the prevention of opportunistic infections.

The most effective way to prevent opportunistic infections is to use effective ART. However, in many patients ART may only be started once severe immune-deficiency has already occurred. Patients may remain immune-deficient even on ART. It is possible to prevent many opportunistic infections in people with low immunity (who have a CD4 cell count below 200 cells / mm^3, or signs of opportunistic infections e.g. oral thrush).

Prophylaxis therapy against some of the common or severe opportunistic infections has had important beneficial effect on the wellbeing and survival of people with HIV/AIDS. The prophylaxis is usually with commonly used medication which may not be too costly.

PRIMARY CARE FOR LATE HIV/AIDS

Drugs may be used to prevent the following common HIV-related infections:

- *Candida albicans* (thrush)
- *Pneumocystis carinii*
- Tuberculosis
- Toxoplasmosis
- Herpes simplex infection
- Bacterial pneumonia
- Cryptococcal meningitis
- Herpes zoster (shingles)
- Others *(see Chapter 7)*

As a general rule, you should consider the prophylactic measures below, when the immune-deficiency is at an advanced stage.

◆ *Candida albicans* prophylaxis (prevention)

Candida (oral and vaginal) commonly starts to appear when the CD4 count drops below 350 cells/mm³. It is a very common opportunistic infection. Candida may spread further into the oesophagus as the immune-deficiency deteriorates.

It is best and cheapest to start with locally applied agents, and after that to give tablets with a systemic effect.

The following is a list of the agents in order of cost and strength. The more expensive agents are usually used for more severe or resistant infections.

Local applications

Apply one of the following:

Chlorhexidene

- This is available in a 0,02% solution.
- Use as a mouthwash, 12 hourly.

Nystatin (Mycostatin)

- 1 – 3 tablets, 8 – 12 hourly
  or
- An oral suspension (1 – 2 ml), 6 hourly

Amphotericin B lozenges (Fungizone)

- ½ lozenge to be sucked, 6 – 12 hourly or more frequently if necessary.

Miconazole gel (Daktarin)

- This is applied 12 – 24 hourly

Systemic medication

Ketoconazole (Nizoral)

- Usually used if the above agents do not clear up the infection.

- Dosage 200 mg daily

- This can be given 12 hourly if:

  - the 200 mg daily dose is not effective

  - there is severe infection

  - there is infection in the oesophagus

- It is best for severe thrush and is often needed in very severe immune-deficiency.

- You may need to use ketoconazole to clear up an infection and thereafter continue with one of the less powerful agents on the previous page.

- Ketoconazole can be toxic to the liver and should be used very carefully if there is any liver disease.

Fluconazole

- Dosage 100 mg daily

- This is a newer agent, less toxic than ketoconazole.

- It can be used in very severe cases.

- Fluconazole is preferred for cryptococcal infections.

Itraconazole

- 100 – 200 mg daily

- Used if other agents do not help at all.

- Avoid in pregnancy and breast feeding.

- Caution in liver disease.

Note: **Vaginal thrush** is also commonly present in women with oral thrush. If vaginal thrush develops, it should be treated with locally applied agents, such as nystatin (Mycostatin), miconazole (Daktarin) or clotrimazole (Canestan). If there is persistent recurrence or resistance to local applications, then systemic agents described above should be used *(see also page 136)*. Treatment for thrush usually has to be ongoing as the thrush may continually recur without prophylaxis.

> **When a patient reaches the stage of more advanced immune-deficiency (CD4 less than 350 cells/mm³) or has any sign of oral or vaginal candida, then you should start candida prophylaxis.**
> **The medication should be provided intermittently or on a continual basis.**

◆ *Pneumocystis carinii* prophylaxis

As a general rule you should use PCP prophylaxis in patients if the following applies:

 The CD4 count drops below 200 cells/mm³

◆ There is a history of a PCP illness

◆ There have been clinical signs of other AIDS-defining diseases *(see pages 104 and 118)*

One of the following may be used:

Co-trimoxazole (trimethoprim-sulphamethoxazole – Bactrim, Septran, Cotrim, Purbac and Ultrazole)

◆ Give 2 tablets daily (or 1 double-strength tablet daily) i.e. 960 mg daily

  – 3 x a week e.g. on Mondays, Wednesdays and Fridays

  – **or** 5 days a week (Monday to Friday)

◆ Co-trimoxazole intolerance (side effects) is common and usually presents with a maculo-papular rash. In mild cases an antihistamine medication may help. In more severe cases the drug should be stopped. There have also been recent reports of increasing bacterial reactions to co-trimoxazole.

◆ Dapsone 100 mg daily can be tried as an alternative to co-trimoxazole.

Alternative options include:

Dapsone

◆ Give 100 mg twice a week (e.g. Monday and Thursday).

Pentamidine (Pentacarinat)

◆ Give 300 mg monthly in an aerosolised suspension. The pentamidine is added to 5 ml sterile water and used with a Respigard mask and nebuliser system. This is a very costly alternative.

Pneumocystis carinii, **a protozoal parasite causing life-threatening pneumonia, usually occurs when there is severe immune-deficiency (CD4 count below 200 cells / mm³). Co-trimoxazole is the preferred choice for PCP prophylaxis.**

◆ Tuberculosis prophylaxis

TB prophylaxis is mainly aimed at preventing re-activation of latent TB bacilli (*see also Chapter 11*).

Prophylaxis against TB is effective but its use is controversial. It may be recommended for selected patients (*see below*). The following is recommended:

Isoniazid (INH)

◆ INH is the drug of choice for prophylaxis therapy for TB. For the average size adult, give 300 mg daily.

◆ Prophylaxis should be continued for at least 9 – 12 months.

◆ It can be started at any time but some clinicians wait for the CD4 cell count to drop below 400 cells / mm^3. It should also be used in HIV-positive individuals who have had recent close contact with open pulmonary TB patients.

◆ Prophylaxis is most effective in individuals who are Mantoux skin positive.

◆ Pyridoxine 25 – 50 mg daily should be given with the INH.

◆ Rifampicin plus pyrazinamide (PZA) given for 2 months is an alternative prophylactic option.

Prophylaxis for TB should only be considered in the following circumstances:

◆ There are **no** signs or symptoms of active TB i.e. unexplained weight loss, cough, sweats at night, chest pains, haemoptysis (coughing blood-stained sputum), clinical signs of chest disease, matted and enlarged lymph nodes. Ideally a chest X-ray should be normal and free of any suggestion of TB.

◆ The patient should:
  – have a record of regular follow-up visits
  – be likely to be compliant with therapy
  – follow the prophylaxis medication properly

◆ The CD4 cell count should be 400 cells / mm^3 or less, or there should be other clinical signs suggestive of immune-deficiency
  – some clinicians advise TB prophylaxis earlier in the stage of the disease.

Note: The co-trimoxazole prophylaxis medication (*see page 109*) has also been shown to reduce the likelihood of death due to TB in a dual HIV-infected patient.

◆ Toxoplasmosis prophylaxis

It is also possible to prevent toxoplasmosis.

You can use one of the following:

Co-trimoxazole (trimethoprim-sulphamethoxazole)

 2 tablets 12 hourly on Mondays, Wednesdays, Fridays
(i.e. 3 times a week)

or

Trimethoprim (Triprim Proloprim) and dapsone

◆ 2 tablets trimethoprim, combined with 100 mg dapsone, twice a week

◆ Severe and recurrent herpes infections

If herpes infection is recurrent, severe and very debilitating, prophylaxis should be considered if affordable.

Valciclovir

◆ 500 mg 12 hourly

Acyclovir

◆ 400 – 800 mg 12 hourly is recommended.

◆ Immunisation against infectious diseases

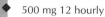 Live vaccines should generally be avoided in adults. Immune-deficient patients (CD4 < 200) frequently have a poor antigenic response to all types of vaccines. There may also be a temporary rise in viral load after a vaccination is given.

The following vaccinations are recommended:

◆ Influenza – annually

◆ Hepatitis B – if the patient is hepatitis B surface antigen negative (especially if the patient is at risk or living in a high hepatitis B prevalence area)

Note:

◆ Yellow fever vaccine can be given if the CD4 cell count is above 200.

◆ Pneumococcal (23 polyvalent) vaccine may be harmful and **should not** be given. Further trials on other Pneumococcal vaccines are being awaited.

◆ Secondary prophylaxis

In some circumstances secondary prophylaxis could be offered to selected patients if:

– resources are available

– the patient is likely to adhere to the therapy

The following conditions are suitable for secondary prophylaxis:

◆ Post cryptococcal meningitis

   – fluconazole 100 – 200 mg daily *(see also table on page 156)*

◆ Post tuberculosis

   – rifampicin, INH, daily Monday to Friday

◆ Oesophageal candidiasis

   – fluconazole, ketoconazole *(see above and page 155)*

◆ Toxoplasmosis

   – *see pages 111 and 156*

◆ Recurrent and severe herpes infection

   – *see pages 111 and 156*

Antimicrobial drug-resistance may result from the unsupervised or erratic use of these drugs. Patients who 'qualify' for antimicrobial preventative therapy must be compliant with treatment. They must also attend the clinic regularly.

◆ Preventing food-borne infection / diarrhoeal disease

Health workers should encourage patients, particularly with very low CD4 counts or signs of immune-deficiency (100 cells / mm^3) to do the following:

◆ Avoid raw (undercooked) meat.

◆ Peel fruit or at least wash it well before eating.

◆ Boil all drinking water in areas where there is unsafe water supply.

The table on the following page summarises the prophylaxis of opportunistic infections.

The general medical examination, investigations, ART and the prevention of some important opportunistic infections have been discussed. Another feature of the management of people with advanced HIV disease is the care and treatment of various opportunistic infections and other HIV-related conditions (see the following pages).

Refer also to the graph in Chapter 5 (on page 94) concerning ART and prophylactic therapy in relation to the CD4 cell count.

◆ Opportunistic infection prophylaxis therapy

The following table outlines the various drug options and dosages etc. for prophylaxis therapy. (Some of the options are unaffordable for many patients, but hopefully more affordable medication will be available in the future.)

Options for prophylactic therapy

Disease to be prevented (pathogen)	Agent	Dosage	Schedule	Indication
Candidiasis (thrush) – oral – oesophageal – genital	See list on pages 135 – 136	See list on pages 135 – 136	See list on pages 135 – 136	◆ Intermittently or continuously after the first appearance of the candidiasis
Reactivation tuberculosis	Isoniazid (INH)	300 mg	Daily with meals for 6 –12 months	◆ CD4 cell count 400 cells / mm^3 ◆ Exclude active TB ◆ Compliant patient
Pneumocystis carinii pneumonia, some bacterial infections, toxoplasma gondii	Co-trimoxazole (Bactrim)	1 or 2 single strength tablets	Daily with meals	◆ CD4 cell count 200 cells / mm^3 – or clinical signs of immune-deficiency
Streptococcus pneumoniae	Pneumococcal polyvalent (23) vaccine	0,5 ml	1M injection (once)	◆ At initial assessment CD4 cell count 200 cells / mm^3
Severe recurrent herpes infection	Valciclovir	500 mg	12 hourly	◆ If recurrent severe infections
	Acyclovir	400 – 800 mg	12 hourly	
Viral influenza	Influenza vaccine	0,5 ml	1M injection annually	◆ CD4 cell count 100 cells / mm^3
Cryptococcus meningitis (secondary prophylaxis)	Fluconazole	100 – 200 mg	Daily with meals	◆ Previous cryptococcal meningitis

See also table on page 155

Treating opportunistic infections and other HIV-related conditions

Advanced HIV disease is associated with various opportunistic infections and other HIV-related conditions

◆ There may be an obvious problem, such as thrush, herpes 'cold sore', dermatitis etc., which can be diagnosed and treated immediately.

◆ The patient may be complaining of an important symptom, such as persistent headache, weight loss, cough, diarrhoea or fever, which needs investigation and treatment. These conditions need to be investigated and managed according to usual medical principles and practices.

◆ You may discover an abnormal finding during examination which needs further investigation and care, such as a localised or generalised lymphadenopathy, an abnormal finding on respiratory examination or an unusual skin condition etc.

You may also need to refer the patient to a specialist or hospital to help make a diagnosis and/or to manage specific medical problems.

As a general rule, most conditions can be managed as usual, as for any patient with or without HIV infection. Use the most simple and cost-effective treatments possible. Some conditions need special or longer care in the HIV positive patient.

The most common HIV-related conditions and their investigation and management are discussed in Chapter 7 and summarised in the table on page 155.

As the disease progresses pain relief and palliative care may be needed (*see Chapter 14*).

Effective ART usually elevates the CD4 cell count, and this in turn can prevent most opportunistic infections.

Support, counselling and referral

It is best to manage people with HIV/AIDS with a team of health workers. The team may include a primary care doctor or nurse, nursing sisters, social workers, psychologists, counsellors, health educators, voluntary workers and specialists.

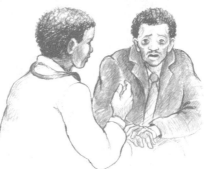

However, in some areas, you may not have a full team and you may find you have to fulfil many of these roles yourself.

People with HIV/AIDS have to cope with many different problems. These problems vary from medical conditions to psycho-social problems, which are often related to coping with the disease and crises, such as anxiety, fear or depression.

- A patient may have feelings of despair, guilt, shame, hopelessness, anger etc.

- Problems may arise as a result of ART, such as drug failure, side effects, toxicity, adherence etc.

- Problems may also be related to their work, their personal relationships, their families and their sexual activity.

- Sleep problems are common and may need to be managed.

- Financial and social problems may arise.

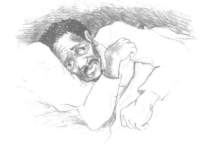

- Problems may also relate to having children, becoming pregnant, and in the prevention of mother to child transmission during pregnancy and infant feeding.

- Fear, anxiety and depression may be related to thoughts of dying, and spiritual support and help may be needed.

The primary caregiver needs to do the following:

◆ Identify the kinds of problems on the previous page and deal with them in the best possible way. You may be able to effectively counsel the patient yourself. You may need to refer the person to a counsellor, such as a social worker or clinical psychologist or to someone specifically experienced in counselling people with HIV/AIDS. *Chapter 13 deals with counselling in more detail.*

◆ Encourage and support your patients. The health worker and the patient should view HIV disease as a chronic manageable condition. It will need monitoring, early medical intervention and close co-operation between health worker and patient.

◆ Promote healthier lifestyles, such as diet, exercise, sleep, smoking-reduction etc. *(see page 94).*

◆ Discuss problems relating to sexual activity and encourage the continuance of safer sexual practices, and even explore ways of enjoying sex in a safe manner *(see page 96).*

◆ Consider referral to other known agencies, such as social welfare organisations, hospice associations, church support groups, community support groups, financial and family aid organisations. There may be community AIDS organisations in your area, specifically set up to support and aid people and families affected by AIDS *(see reference on page 98).*

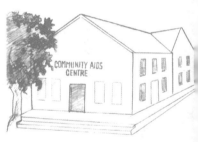

◆ You may also need to see and counsel the wife, husband or partner, a close relative or friend, a child or employer (with the patient's consent).

Counselling is discussed in more detail in Chapter 13, and managing people who are dying in Chapter 14.

Remember the psychological, mental and social support and care of people with HIV/AIDS is as important as their medical management.

Home-care, day-care, hospital or hospice

As the patient's condition deteriorates, problems may arise in keeping the patient at home.

At this stage you may need to consider arranging visits to his/her home by a community nurse. Alternatively day-care centres or hospice organisations may be available. Hospital care is expensive and should only be used for the care of medical problems or if other forms of community care are not available.

Aspects of the management of people in the terminal stages of HIV disease are discussed in Chapter 14.

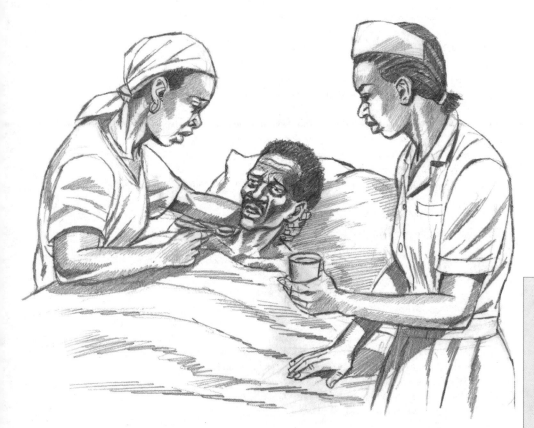

The management of specific HIV-related medical conditions is discussed in the next chapter.

World Health Organisation Staging System for HIV Infection and Disease

CLINICAL STAGE 1

1. Acute retroviral infection
2. Asymptomatic
3. Persistent generalised lymphadenopathy (enlargement of the lymph nodes)

    Performance scale 1: asymptomatic, normal activity

CLINICAL STAGE 2

4. Weight loss, <10% of body weight
5. Minor mucocutaneous manifestations (seborrhoeic dermatitis, prurigo (chronic itchy skin), fungal nail infections, recurrent oral ulcerations, angular cheilitis (inflammation of the corners of the mouth)
6. Herpes zoster (shingles), within the last 5 years
7. Recurrent upper respiratory tract infections (i.e. bacterial sinusitis)

    And/or performance scale 2: symptomatic, normal activity

CLINICAL STAGE 3

8. Weight loss, >10% of body weight
9. Unexplained chronic diarrhoea, >1 month
10. Unexplained prolonged fever (intermittent or constant), >1 month
11. Oral candidiasis (thrush)
12. Vulvo-vaginal candidiasis, chronic (>1 month) or poorly responsive to therapy
13. Oral hairy leukoplakia (thickening of the dorsal surface of the tongue)
14. Pulmonary tuberculosis, within the past year
15. Severe bacterial infections (e.g. pneumonia)

    And / or performance scale 3: bedridden <50% of the day during the last month

CLINICAL STAGE 4 (AIDS-defining conditions)

16. HIV wasting syndrome, as defined
17. *Pneumocystis carinii* pneumonia
18. Toxoplasmosis of an internal organ
19. Cryptosporidiosis with diarrhoea, >1 month
20. Cryptosporidiosis, extrapulmonary
21. Cytomegalovirus (disease of an organ other than liver, spleen or lymph nodes)
22. Herpes simplex virus infection, mucocutaneous >1 month, or visceral (any duration)
23. Progressive multifocal leuko-encephalopathy (selective destruction of the central nervous system)
24. Any disseminated endemic mycosis (i.e. histoplasmosis, coccidioidomycosis)
25. Candidiasis of the oesophagus, trachea, bronchi or lungs
26. Atypical mycobacteriosis, disseminated
27. Non-typhoid salmonella septicaemia
28. Extrapulmonary tuberculosis
29. Lymphoma
30. Kaposi's sarcoma
31. HIV encephalopathy or dementia as defined

    And / or performance scale 4: bedridden >50% of the day during the last month

The Center for Disease Control (USA) case definition of AIDS

Acquired immuno-deficiency syndrome (AIDS) is an aggregate of signs and symptoms and illnesses resulting from a compromised immune system. A diagnosis of AIDS requires the definitive or presumptive diagnosis of one or more 'indicator diseases' and, depending on certain criteria, may or may not require laboratory evidence of HIV infection. The following outline is used by physicians in the United States to arrive at an AIDS diagnosis.

I A diagnosis of AIDS can be made if laboratory evidence of HIV infection has been established and a definitive diagnosis of any of the following indicator diseases has been made – regardless of the presence of other causes of immuno-deficiency.

- ◆ Adolescents and adults with CD4 and lymphocyte counts less than 200 cells/mm³
- ◆ Candidiasis of the oesophagus, trachea, bronchi or lungs
- ◆ Coccidioidomycosis, disseminated (extrapulmonary)
- ◆ Cryptococcosis (extrapulmonary)
- ◆ Cryptosporidiosis with diarrhoea persisting more than 1 month
- ◆ Cytomegalovirus disease of an organ other than the liver, spleen or lymph nodes in a patient older than 1 month
- ◆ Herpes simplex virus infection causing a mucocutaneous ulcer (e.g. in eyes, nose, mouth, and genito anal areas) that persists for more than 1 month; or bronchitis, pneumonitis or oesophagitis caused by herpes simplex virus in a patient older than 1 month
- ◆ Histoplasmosis, disseminated (extrapulmonary)
- ◆ HIV encephalopathy; also called subacute encephalopathy due to HIV; also referred to as HIV dementia or AIDS dementia complex (ADC), which is clinically defined as a disabling cognitive or motor dysfunction interfering with the patient's occupation or activities of daily living, or loss of behavioural developmental milestones in the absence of a concurrent illness or condition
- ◆ HIV wasting syndrome, defined as involuntary weight loss of greater than 10% of body weight plus chronic diarrhoea or chronic weakness and fever in the absence of a concurrent illness or condition; also referred to as 'Slims disease'
- ◆ Isosporiasis with diarrhoea persisting for longer than 1 month
- ◆ Kaposi's sarcoma
- ◆ Lymphoma (primary) of the brain
- ◆ Lymphoid interstitial pneumonitis (LIP) and/or pulmonary lymphoid hyperplasia affecting a child under 13 years of age
- ◆ Mycobacterial disease including pulmonary infection, disseminated and extrapulmonary *Mycobacterium tuberculosis* disease
- ◆ *Mycobacterium avium,* disseminated
- ◆ Non-Hodgkin's lymphoma
- ◆ *Pneumocystis carinii* pneumonia
- ◆ Progressive multifocal leukoencephalopathy
- ◆ Salmonella septicaemia, recurrent
- ◆ Toxoplasmosis of the brain
- ◆ Strongyloidosis extrainterstitial
- ◆ Any combination of at least two of the following bacterial infections within a 2 year period affecting a patient less than 13 years of age: septicaemia, pneumonia, meningitis, bone or joint infection, or abscess of an internal organ or body cavity caused by haemophilus, streptococcus or other fever-inducing bacteria
- ◆ Recurrent pneumonia
- ◆ Invasive cervical cancer

II A diagnosis of AIDS can be made if laboratory evidence of HIV is positive and any of the following indicator diseases is diagnosed presumptively. (A presumptive diagnosis is generally made in situations in which the patient's condition does not permit the performance of definitive testing.)

◆ Candidiasis of the oesophagus

◆ Cytomegalovirus retinitis with loss of vision

◆ Kaposi's sarcoma

◆ Lymphoid interstitial pneumonitis and/or pulmonary lymphoid hyperplasia affecting a patient less than 13 years of age

◆ Mycobacterial disease, disseminated

◆ *Pneumocystis carinii* pneumonia

◆ Toxoplasmosis of the brain in a patient older than 1 month

III A diagnosis of AIDS can be made if laboratory evidence of HIV infection is *lacking* or *inconclusive* **but** a definitive diagnosis of any of the following indicator diseases is made, provided other known causes of immuno-deficiency are ruled out.

◆ Candidiasis of the oesophagus, trachea, bronchi, or lungs

◆ Cryptococcosis, extrapulmonary

◆ Cryptosporidiosis with diarrhoea persisting longer than 1 month

◆ Cytomegalovirus disease of an organ other than the liver, spleen, or lymph nodes in a patient older than 1 month

◆ Herpes simplex virus infection causing a mucocutaneous ulcer that persists longer than 1 month; or bronchitis, pneumonitis or oesophagitis affecting a patient older than 1 month

◆ Kaposi's sarcoma affecting a patient below 60 years of age

◆ Lymphoma of the brain (primary) affecting a patient less than 60 years of age

◆ Lymphoid interstitial pneumonitis and/or pulmonary lymphoid hyperplasia affecting a patient less than 13 years of age

◆ *Mycobacterium avium* complex or *Mycobacterium kansasii* disease, disseminated

◆ *Pneumocystis carinii* pneumonia

◆ Progressive multifocal leukoencephalopathy

◆ Toxoplasmosis of the brain in a patient older than 1 month

IV A diagnosis of AIDS can also be made when laboratory evidence of HIV infection is negative. If all other causes of immuno-deficiency are excluded and the patient has had either a definitive diagnosis of *Pneumocystis carinii* pneumonia or a definitive diagnosis of any of the indicator diseases of AIDS and a CD4 (T4) cell count less than 400 cells/mm³.

Correlation of HIV-related diseases / conditions with CD4 cell counts

(See Archives of Internal Medicine 1995;155;1537)

CD4 cell count*	Infections	Non-infectious+
> 500 / mm³	Acute retroviral syndrome; Candidal vaginitis	Persistent generalised lymphadenopathy (PGL); Guillain-Barré syndrome; Myopathy; Aseptic meningitis
200 – 500 / mm³	Pneumococcal and bacterial pneumonia; Pulmonary TB; Herpes zoster; Oral, pharyngeal and sometimes oesophageal candidiasis (thrush); Cryptosporidiosis – (self-limited); Kaposi's sarcoma; Oral hairy leukoplakia	Cervical intraepithelial neoplasia; Cervical cancer; B-cell lymphoma; Anaemia; Mononeuronal multiplex; Idiopathic thrombocytopaenic purpura; Hodgkin's lymphoma; Lymphocytic interstitial pneumonitis
< 200 / mm³ (commonly associated with a lymphocyte count of 1 200 / ml or less)	*P. carinii* pneumonia; Disseminated / chronic Herpes simplex; Toxoplasmosis; Cryptococcosis; Disseminated histoplasmosis and coccidioidomycosis; Microsporidiosis; Miliary/extrapulmonary TB; Progressive multifocal leukoencephalopathy (PML); Candidal oesophagitis	Wasting; Peripheral neuropathy; HIV-associated dementia; CNS lymphoma; Cardiomyopathy; Vacuolar myelopathy; Progressive polyradiculopathy; Immunoblastic lymphoma
< 50 / mm³	Disseminated CMV; Disseminated *M. avium* complex	

* Most complications occur with increased frequency at lower CD4 counts.
+ Some conditions listed as 'non-infectious' are probably associated with transmissible microbes e.g. lymphoma (EBV) and cervical cancer (HPV).

PRIMARY CARE FOR LATE HIV/AIDS

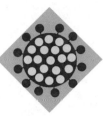

Chapter 7

GUIDELINES FOR RECOGNISING AND MANAGING COMMON AND IMPORTANT HIV-ASSOCIATED CONDITIONS

Respiratory conditions

Diarrhoeal disease

Candidiasis

Hairy leukoplakia (Epstein-Barr virus)

Skin conditions

Malignancy

Lymphadenopathy

Headache

Neurological disease

Cytomegalovirus (CMV) retinal infection

Toxoplasmosis

Fever (pyrexia)

Weight loss

Treatment and secondary prophylaxis of opportunistic infections in adults

People with HIV infection are susceptible to a large variety of different conditions and medical problems. This chapter will outline some of the most common and important conditions which may present to the primary care clinician.

Respiratory conditions

Respiratory infections are common in advanced HIV disease.

◆ Common symptoms

Cough, dyspnoea, fever, night sweats, weight loss and tachypnoea are suggestive of respiratory infection.

The following are the most common respiratory infections:

Acute onset of symptoms (1 – 5 days) think of:

- Bacterial infections e.g. *Haemophilus influenzae*, streptococcal, pneumococcal, *Staphylococcus aureus*
- Atypical pneumonia (mycoplasma)

Note: TB can also start acutely in severely immune-deficient patients.

Chronic onset of symptoms (2 – 4 weeks or more) think of:

- *Mycobacterium tuberculosis*
- *Pneumocystis carinii* pneumonia
- Viral pneumonia (cytomegalovirus)
- Fungal pneumonia (cryptococcus, histoplasmosis, coccidioidomycosis)
- Toxoplasma pneumonia

Other conditions which may cause respiratory symptoms and signs include Kaposi's sarcoma and lymphoma.

See Chapter 11 for details on tuberculosis.

◆ Investigations

Sputum examination

Sputum examination is helpful and should include a gram stain, an acid fast bacilli examination, a culture and fungal studies.

- Green/yellow sputum may indicate acute bacterial infection.
- Sputum can also be examined in the laboratory for pneumocystic and fungal infections.
- Acid fast bacilli on microscopy or culture will help to diagnose TB infection.

Chest X-ray

Chest X-ray is often helpful. Patients with immune-deficiency may develop typical or unusual X-ray changes.

◆ Effusions/cavities may indicate tuberculosis.

◆ Bilateral interstitial infiltrates may indicate *Pneumocystis carinii*.

◆ Lobar consolidation is typical of acute bacterial infection (and may also indicate tuberculosis with HIV infection).

Bronchoscopy

Bronchoscopy can be used, if available, if there is no response to initial treatment or if the diagnosis is doubtful. It is usually only available in larger hospitals and in the bigger towns and cities.

Bronchoscopy and laboratory examination of bronchoscopic fluids are especially helpful in diagnosing the following:

◆ *Pneumocystis carinii*

◆ Fungal infection

◆ Toxoplasmosis

◆ Viral pneumonia

◆ Some of the tumours
e.g. Kaposi's sarcoma and lymphoma

Pneumonia is common and often the first 'serious' opportunistic infection the patient experiences.

◆ Many pneumonias are due to common gram-positive and negative organisms and sometimes mycoplasma pneumonia.

◆ However atypical forms of pneumonia, and pneumonia due to TB, PCP, viruses and fungi, may be difficult to definitively diagnose. Clinicians need to be highly aware of these forms of infection.

◆ Tuberculosis should always be considered as it may present in unusual or atypical ways.

◆ Acute respiratory infection – pneumonia

Treatment

R_x

Unless a specific bacteria is isolated, and antibiotic sensitivities are available, treatment should generally be commenced with:

◆ Amoxicillin / ampicillin, penicillin, Augmentin or tetracyclines may be considered for initial therapy. Co-trimoxazole is a useful first-line antibiotic as it is effective against many bacteria, mycoplasma and *Pneumocystis carinii* infection.

◆ For more complicated infections, or for infections not responsive to the above, consider:

– a cephalosporin orally or parentally

– a macrolide (erythromycin, roxithromycin etc.)

Refer very ill patients to a hospital.

Therapy for TB or for PCP should be considered if the patient remains unresponsive to the above options, or if the clinical picture is strongly suggestive of these conditions.

See also pages 155 – 156.

◆ Chronic respiratory infection

Tuberculosis

Tuberculosis is the most common cause of chronic pneumonia in developing countries. Remember that TB can also have a more acute onset, especially in severely immune-deficient patients. TB is usually associated with CD4 cell counts less than 350 cells/mm³. TB is discussed in detail in *Chapter 11*. Use the regular TB treatment regimes.

See page 254 for a discussion on ART and TB.

Directly Observed Therapy (DOT)

◆ The best way to ensure that a TB patient completes TB treatment is with Directly Observed Therapy (DOT).

◆ TB treatment is generally the same for HIV-positive or negative people.

Treatment regimens are given on the next page, and these should be reviewed and kept updated with national guidelines for TB treatment.

Note:

◆ Treatment is given 5 days a week in the intensive phase i.e.

– the first 2 months of treatment in new patients;

– and the first 3 months of treatment in re-treatment patients.

◆ Hospitalised TB patients can receive the same dosages 7 days per week.

◆ For the continuation phase, treatment is given 5 days a week i.e.

– the last 4 months of treatment for new patients

– and the last 5 months of treatment for re-treatment patients.

Recommended TB treatment regimens

◆ Adult patients (Regimen 1)

New smear or culture-positive and other serious pulmonary and extrapulmonary tuberculosis

Pre-treatment body weight	2 months Initial Phase (treatment given 5 times a week)	4 months Continuation Phase (treatment given 5 times a week)	
	Combination tablet RHZE 120 / 60 / 300 / 200 mg*	Combination tablet RH 150 / 100 mg	Combination tablet RH 300 / 150 mg
< 50 kg	4 tabs	3 tabs	
> 50 kg	5 tabs		2 tabs
*Ethambutol 225 mg in combination is also acceptable			

◆ Re-treatment adult patients (Regimen 2)

Smear or culture positive re-treatment cases

Pre-treatment body weight	2 months Initial Phase (treatment given 5 times a week)		3rd month (5 times a week)	5 months Continuation Phase (5 times a week)			
	RHZE 120 / 60 / 300 / 200 mg*	Streptomycin	RHZE	RH 150 / 100 mg	E 400 mg	RH 300 / 150 mg	E 400 mg
< 50 kg	4 tabs	750 mg	4 tabs	3 tabs	2 tabs		
> 50 kg	5 tabs	1 000 mg	5 tabs			2 tabs	3 tabs

Note: Streptomycin (S) is given by intramuscular injection. It should be reduced to 750 mg per day to those older than 45 years, and not be given to those over 65 years.
*Ethambutol 225 mg in combination is also acceptable.

*R = rifampicin; H = isoniazid (INH); Z = pyrazinamide; E = ethambutol; S= streptomycin

If the combination drugs are not available, the treatment plan on the previous page can be used with the following drugs and their dosages:		
Drug name	**Under 50 kg body wt**	**Over 50 kg body wt**
Rifampicin	450 mg daily	600 mg daily
INH	300 mg daily	300 mg daily
Pyrazinamide	1 000 mg daily	1 500 mg daily
Ethambutol	800 mg daiy	1 200 mg daily

Multi drug-resistant TB (MDR)

Multi drug-resistant TB (MDR) refers to TB which is resistant to isoniazid and rifampicin. MDR is difficult and expensive to treat. Currently, the cure rate of MDR patients is less than 50%. It is therefore essential to prevent the development of MDR (*see page 257*).

MDR is diagnosed by TB culture and susceptibility testing. Refer MDR patients to a MDR unit where experienced clinicians can treat the patient.

Pneumocystis carinii (PC) and Pneumocystis carinii pneumonia (PCP)

This infection is relatively common in patients with immune-deficiency. It usually occurs in the more severely immune-deficient individual, e.g. CD4 levels below 200 cells / mm^3, but it may also occur at higher levels.

PCP can be difficult to diagnose. It can progress rapidly to a severe and life-threatening pneumonia. For this reason it may be necessary to treat for PCP infection on clinical suspicion alone, or if there is any doubt about the diagnosis.

Consider PCP if there are:

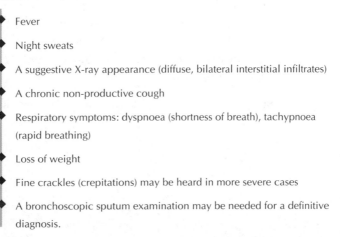

- Fever

- Night sweats

- A suggestive X-ray appearance (diffuse, bilateral interstitial infiltrates)

- A chronic non-productive cough

- Respiratory symptoms: dyspnoea (shortness of breath), tachypnoea (rapid breathing)

- Loss of weight

- Fine crackles (crepitations) may be heard in more severe cases

- A bronchoscopic sputum examination may be needed for a definitive diagnosis.

Treatment

℞

Mild and moderate cases could probably be treated with oral co-trimoxazole (Bactrim) and more severe cases should be treated in hospital. These patients will require intravenous co-trimoxazole (Bactrim) and steroids.

Mild to moderate PCP

◆ Co-trimoxazole e.g. Bactrim, Septran, Purbac, Trib 2 DS (double-strength) tablets or 4 SS (single-strength) tablets 4 x daily after meals for 14 – 21 days

◆ Alternative options are:

  – dapsone 100 mg plus trimethoprim 300 mg 8 hourly

  – clindamycin 600 mg 4 x daily plus pyrimethamine 50 mg daily *(see also table page 156)*

Moderate to severe PCP

◆ Co-trimoxazole (Bactrim) 15 – 20 mg / kg trimethoprim component

  – this should be divided into 6 hourly doses per day

◆ Prednisone 40 mg 2 x daily after meals for 5 days

  – then prednisone 20 mg daily after meals for 14 days

◆ Oxygen therapy if there is poor oxygenation of the blood.

◆ Consider referral of patient to a larger centre.

◆ Dapsone 100 mg daily with trimethoprim 200 mg 8 hourly can also be used if there is allergy to the co-trimoxazole (i.e. leaving out the sulphamethoxazole component)

See also table on page 155.

◆ Other respiratory infections and conditions

Other infections, such as fungi, viral, toxoplasmosis, Kaposi's sarcoma etc., are difficult to diagnose. They usually require special diagnostic facilities (bronchoscopy and / or biopsy) and other laboratory techniques. Antifungal and antiviral medication is usually expensive and should be used by experienced clinicians.

Note: Chest physiotherapy is also helpful for most respiratory infections.

Diarrhoeal disease

Diarrhoea usually occurs at some stage in most people with advanced HIV disease. The diarrhoea can be very distressing and may seriously disturb the patient's daily life. It is often ongoing and may result in serious dehydration and/or electrolyte loss. Weight loss also commonly accompanies the ongoing diarrhoea.

The onset of persistent diarrhoea often indicates severe immune-deficiency with a poor prognosis.

◆ Bacteria are common pathogens.

◆ In more advanced immune-deficiency, fungal (cryptosporidium, isospora, giardia, microsporidia) and viral infection viruses (herpes, CMV) are common.

◆ Amoebiasis and giardia may be other causes.

◆ It is often difficult to isolate the specific cause of the diarrhoea.

◆ Diarrhoea in people with immune-deficiency is often difficult to treat and to control.

The therapeutic approach to diarrhoea includes:

◆ Maintaining or correcting hydration and electrolyte loss

◆ Investigating and treating the cause

◆ Anti-diarrhoeal agents

◆ Diet/food supplements

See also table page 156.

◆ Maintaining or correcting hydration and electrolyte loss

Hydration maintenance

Look for signs of dehydration, such as a rapid pulse, dry mouth, sunken eyes, poor skin elasticity, poor urine output and in severe cases even confusion or loss of consciousness.

Oral fluids, soups etc. should be taken frequently during the day.

A good home-made oral hydration fluid:

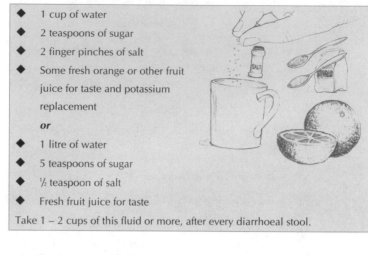

- ◆ 1 cup of water
- ◆ 2 teaspoons of sugar
- ◆ 2 finger pinches of salt
- ◆ Some fresh orange or other fruit juice for taste and potassium replacement

or

- ◆ 1 litre of water
- ◆ 5 teaspoons of sugar
- ◆ ½ teaspoon of salt
- ◆ Fresh fruit juice for taste

Take 1 – 2 cups of this fluid or more, after every diarrhoeal stool.

N.B. Give intravenous fluids for marked dehydration.

Electrolyte replacement

Potassium and sodium are usually lost in the diarrhoea and need to be replaced. The oral hydration fluid will usually replace most of the sodium. It is often necessary to replace the potassium with potassium supplements, such as Slow K, given 6 – 12 hourly.

In severe or ongoing diarrhoea you may need to replace other essential elements, such as magnesium, calcium etc. Monitoring the blood electrolyte and albumin level is usually necessary in people with chronic diarrhoea.

◆ Investigating and treating the cause

Investigating the cause of the diarrhoea in the primary care setting may be difficult and is often unsuccessful. Causes of diarrhoea may differ in different areas.

Guide to symptoms and possible cause of diarrhoea

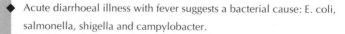

- ◆ Acute diarrhoeal illness with fever suggests a bacterial cause: E. coli, salmonella, shigella and campylobacter.

- ◆ Parasites, such as cryptosporidium, isospora, giardia, microsporidia and strongyloides, are more likely to cause chronic diarrhoea with minimal generalised body effects.

- ◆ Chronic, re-occuring diarrhoea with minimal symptoms in patients with advanced immune-deficiency (AIDS) suggests cryptosporidiosis or microsporidiosis.

- Abdominal pain, discomfort and / or bloody diarrhoea suggests CMV colitis.

- Diarrhoea may also be part of a systemic illness like disseminated tuberculosis (TB), Mycobacterium avium-intracellulare (MAI), cytomegalovirus, herpes and adenovirus infections.

- CMV colitis causes fever, weight loss and diarrhoea:

    - the diarrhoea may be bloody

    - abdominal pain and cramps are often persistent, severe and debilitating

    - ART may be effective for the prevention and the treatment of CMV-related disease – however this form of therapy is not usually available in public health services.

Persistant diarrhoeal disease may need:

- A full microbiological investigation (stool microscopy, cultures etc.)

- A sigmoidoscopy / colonoscopy with biopsy in severe cases.

Treatment

> **The following drugs can be used as first-line treatment:**
>
> - Co-trimoxazole (Bactrim, Septran etc.) is useful against bacterial infection and some of the parasitic infections, such as isospora.
>   Give 2 tablets 12 hourly for a minimum of 5 days. Continue for 3 weeks if there has been no response after 5 – 7 days and if the diagnosis of bacterial diarrhoea is certain.
> - Erythromycin 500 mg 6 hourly for 5 days can be used for campylobacter infection.
> - Metronidazole 200 – 400 mg 8 hourly for 7 days is useful against some of the parasites, such as giardia and entamoeba infection.
> - Anti-helmintics, such as thiabendazole (Mintezol), mebendazole (Vermox), niclosamide (Yomesan), pyrantel pamoate (Combantrin) and albendazole (Zentel), should be used for worm infestation.

◆ Anti-diarrhoeal agents

These may be useful and may help the patient cope with daily life.
See the following page.

℞

The following drugs are commonly used:

◆ Codeine phosphate 10 mg, 6 – 8 hourly

◆ Loperamide (Imodium) 4 mg stat, then 2 mg after each stool
   (maximum up to 16 mg/24 hours)

◆ Diphenoxylate (Lomotil) 2,5 – 5 mg, 6 – 8 hourly

◆ Kaolin-pectin preparations can also be tried

Note: Anti-diarrhoeal drugs should not be used in the presence of
bloody diarrhoea.

◆ Diet / food supplements

℞

◆ The patient with diarrhoea should drink lots of fluids and keep
   well hydrated.

◆ Eat high-energy, soft foods, such as peeled potatoes, rice and porridge.
   Fats such as oil and margarine are also helpful.

◆ Take vitamin and mineral supplements if the diarrhoea is ongoing.

◆ Also take high protein and energy supplements, such as Complan,
   Ensure or PVM, if available.

◆ Avoid high roughage foods, such as grains, fruit peels and green
   vegetables.

Candidiasis

◆ Oesophageal candidiasis

This commonly occurs with severe immune-deficiency. It is usually associated with
CD4 cell counts of 100 or less. It is an AIDS-defining condition.

Symptoms may include:

◆ Difficulty with swallowing

◆ Regurgitation of thick white mucous-like material

◆ Pain on swallowing (dysphagia)

◆ Burning central chest pain especially associated with
   eating

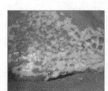

*Oral thrush on upper
palate / uvula and
entering pharynx*

Treatment

℞ Systemic anti-fungals are required. However these are costly and not always available in clinics.

The following should be considered:

◆ Ketoconazole 200 mg daily after meals for 14 days.

◆ **Or** fluconazole 100 mg daily after meals for 10 – 14 days.

◆ Referral to a specialist centre may be necessary.

◆ Oral thrush

Oral thrush is common and one of the first signs of the development of immune-deficiency. It is almost always associated with a low CD4 count (less than 350 cells/mm³).

It usually presents with white plaques on the tongue, palate or inner cheek. They are easily seen and are diagnostic of oral thrush.

In advanced immune-deficiency, the candida infection can spread into the oesophagus and trachea. This may cause difficult or painful swallowing.

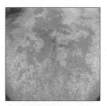
Candidiasis on tongue

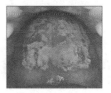
*Oral thrush –
upper palate*

Treatment

℞

The following medication can be used for oral thrush:

◆ Local application of gentian violet 1% aqueous solution.
Apply 8 – 12 hourly

◆ Chlorhexidine 0,02% solution, 12 hourly

◆ Nystatin (Mycostatin) tablets or oral suspension. Suck 1 – 2 tablets, 8 – 12 hourly, or apply 2 – 3 mls of the suspension, 6 – 8 hourly

◆ Amphotericin B lozenges (Fungizone) can be sucked, 12 – 24 hourly or more frequently if necessary

If the above do not clear the thrush then consider:

◆ Clotrimazole (Canestan) solution or miconazole (Daktarin) gel as local applications

In severe infection or in very advanced immune-deficiency or for oesophageal infection you can use the following if available:

◆ Ketoconazole (Nizoral) 200 mg, 12 – 24 hourly orally for 7 – 14 days. It can be toxic to the liver, so use with care in patients with liver problems.

◆ Fluconazole 150 – 200 mg daily for 7 – 14 days

◆ Itraconazole can also be used.
(see also table on page 155)

Once oral thrush has appeared, it is advisable to consider giving prophylaxis therapy, even after the first infection has cleared *(see page 107)*.

Once oral thrush has appeared, it usually means that the immune status is low and other infections, such as TB, *Pneumocystis carinii*, herpes etc., can be expected. Prophylaxis for pneumocystis and TB should be considered *(see pages 109 – 110)*.

◆ Vaginal thrush

Recurrrent or persistent vaginal thrush is another common infection in advanced immune-deficiency.

It usually presents on the labia of the vulvae and in the vagina or on the uppermost skin of the thigh.

Mild vaginal discharge and itching are common symptoms. White plaques may be seen on the vaginal walls and on the inner parts of the labia.

Antibiotics, such as penicillin, tetracycline, erythromycin etc., may destroy the natural vaginal flora and promote the development of thrush. This may occur in healthy (non-HIV-infected) people as well.

Balanitis (thrush of the glans of the penis) is much less common than vulvo-vaginal thrush, and is usually indicative of advanced immune-deficiency.

Treatment

R_x

Treat vaginal thrush as usual.

Use the following in order of severity:

◆ Mycostatin vaginal tablets or cream. Apply 12 hourly

For more severe infection use:

◆ Clotrimazole (Canestan) vaginal tablets or cream.
Apply nightly (may need to be repeated for several nights until symptoms disappear)
or

◆ Miconazole (Daktarin) vaginal tablets/cream.
Apply 12 – 24 hourly for 7 – 14 days
or

◆ Tioconazole (Gyno-trosyd) vaginal tablets/cream.
Apply nightly for 3 – 5 nights

For severe infection use:

◆ Ketoconazole (Nizarol) for severe cases. Take the oral preparation as discussed above or the vaginal tablets nightly for 3 – 5 nights.
or

◆ Fluconazole 150 mg stat

Note: You may have to give the above preparations for longer periods in advanced immune-deficiency.

> **Thrush is a common manifestation of advanced immune-deficiency. Prophylaxis against thrush is an important feature of managing people with advanced HIV disease.**

Hairy leukoplakia (Epstein-Barr virus)

Oral hairy leukoplakia (OHL)

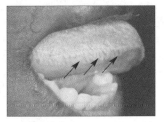

◆ This presents as a white discolouration on the surface and side walls of the tongue.

◆ It often has the appearance of white, thread-like lesions.

◆ It is asymptomatic and the white "patches" cannot be scraped off, nor does the lesion bleed on contact.

Hairy leukoplakia on side of tongue

Treatment

Rₓ

◆ Gentle and regular brushing of the tongue with a soft toothbrush is suggested.

◆ Specific treatment is not recommended as the condition does not usually cause any specific ill effects.

Skin conditions

Skin conditions are common in people with HIV infection. Non-specific conditions may have commenced earlier, before any other symptoms have appeared. Some conditions, such as Herpes zoster (shingles) or Kaposi's sarcoma, occur with advanced HIV infection and are associated with low CD4 counts.

℞

The following is a list of the more common HIV-associated skin conditions:

◆ **Viral infections**

Herpes simplex

Herpes zoster

Molluscum contagiosum

Condylomata acuminata

◆ **Bacterial infections**

Folliculitis (very common)

Furunculosis

Impetigo and other pyoderma (due to staphylococci and streptococci)

◆ **Fungal infections**

Candidiasis

Tinea

◆ **Malignancy**

Kaposi's sarcoma

Other HIV-related skin conditions

Seborrhoeic dermatitis (very common)

Drug eruptions

Urticaria and pruritis

Erythroderma

Psoriasis

Dry, itchy skin

Note: Sexually transmitted infections, such as syphilis, chancroid, Herpes etc., may also be present and may need more prolonged therapy. Peri-anal conditions, such as abscesses, fistulae and dermatitis, may also present as skin problems.

As a general rule, manage skin problems as usual. Some conditions may need longer treatment or you may need to try other medications.

◆ Recognising and treating the common skin conditions

Below are some recommended treatment protocols for some common skin conditions:

Viral infections

Treatment for herpes simplex:

You may find one large blister or ulcer-like lesion e.g. on the lip (cold sore). You may also find multiple, deep or superficial lesions elsewhere on the body and the genitals (these may look like ulcers or blisters/vesicles).

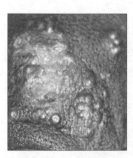

Genital herpes simplex

R_x

Local care:

◆ Keep lesions clean with soap and water.

◆ Topical antiseptic agents are useful, such as 1% gentian violet or chlorhexidine (Hibitane), applied 8 hourly.

◆ Antibiotics and Eusol / betadine dressings may be needed if the lesions become infected.

Specific care:

The following is recommended for severe, resistant or recurrent infections:

◆ Valciclovir 200 – 800 mg, 2 – 3 times daily for 7 days

◆ Acyclovir (Zovirax) 200 mg, 5 times daily for 7 – 10 days (15 – 30 mg/kg/day in children).

However, these drugs are expensive and may not be available for some patients.

◆ Famciclovir 250 mg 3 times daily for 7 – 10 days.

See also page 156.

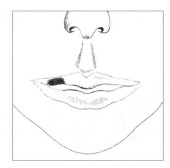

Herpes cold sore

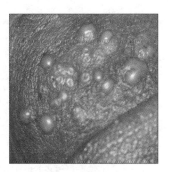

Genital herpes

Treatment for Herpes zoster (shingles)

℞

Local care:
◆ See under herpes simplex *(previous page)*.
Specific care:
◆ Valciclovir (500 mg – 1 g) 3 x daily for
  7 – 10 days
◆ Acyclovir can be used, especially if the
  shingles are widespread or involving the
  face or eye. Give 200 – 400 mg 5 times
  daily for 5 – 10 days.
◆ Shingles is painful and pain relief should
  be offered. Occasionally severe pain
  may be present during or after the lesions
  have healed (post-herpetic neuralgia).
  This can be treated with:
  – amitryptiline (Tryptanol) 25 – 50 mg
    orally daily if the pain is severe
    (see also page 301)
  – consider a short course of oral
    prednisone (10 days)
  See also page 156

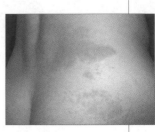

*Herpes zoster
on buttocks*

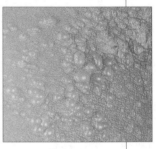

Zoster rash typical

**Remember the onset of Herpes zoster infection usually means
that the HIV infection is in an advanced stage, associated with
low CD4 counts and the likely development of other opportunistic infections.**

Treatment of molluscum contagiosum

Treatment is only necessary for symptomatic lesions or for cosmetic reasons.

℞

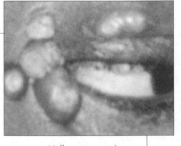

*Molluscum contagiosum
lesions on eye lid*

Local care:
◆ You can prick each lesion with a
  needle or a sharpened orange
  stick which has been dipped in
  phenol.
  This is to express the central core.
◆ Cryotherapy with liquid nitrogen
  is also effective.

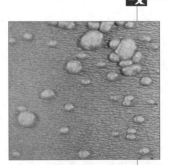

Molluscum contagiosum

Treatment for condylomata acuminata

- ◆ You can treat with podophyllin 20% solution. Paint on and wash off after 6 hours. Repeat 12 hourly for 3 days.
- ◆ You can also use liquid nitrogen, if available. Apply topically and repeat weekly until healed.
- ◆ Extensive lesions need surgical excision.

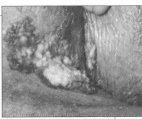

Condylomata acuminata

Bacterial infections

Treatment

- ◆ Other skin infections, such as furunculosis, impetigo etc., need to be treated with systemic antibiotics. Commonly used antibiotics include penicillin, ampicillin, amoxycillin, Augmentin, cloxacillin, tetracycline and erythromycin. A swab for bacterial culture may be necessary, expecially if there is no response to treatment.
- ◆ In severe infection, intravenous therapy may be needed.
- ◆ Surgical drainage is usually required for abscesses.

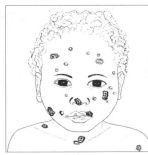

Impetigo

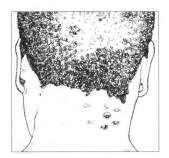

Furunculosis

Folliculitis

Folliculitis is very common. It may present with a fine rash like 'goose-flesh', itching, or a red paular or acne-like lesion.

Treatment

℞

- Regular use of antiseptic lotions (e.g. Hibiscrub).

- 2% sulphur cream applied 3 x daily topically.

- Consider a course of antibiotics, e.g. tetracyclines or cloxacillin if staphalococcal infection is suspected.

- Hydrocortisone cream (or stronger steroid cream) applied 2 x daily may also be useful.

If treatment is ineffective, and if the condition is causing severe symptoms, especially severe itching, then refer to a specialist unit.

Folliculitis

Fungal infections

Tinea infections are common and occur frequently. These infections may be found on the feet, groin, axilla, neck, chest, abdomen, extremities, scalp etc.

Treatment

℞

- Topical antifungal creams, such as Whitfield's ointment, 2 % sulphur cream, clotrimazole (Canestan), miconazole (Daktarin), econazole (Pevaryl), tioconazole (Trosyd), miconazole applied 8 – 12 hourly for 10 – 21 days, are usually effective.

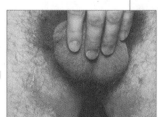

Fungal groin infection

- Oral agents, such as ketoconazole (Nizoral) 200 mg daily for 2 – 3 weeks, can be used in severe or resistant infection.

- Griseofulvin 500 mg orally for 8 – 12 weeks can be taken for a nail infection.

- Selsun and ketoconazole shampoo can be used for a scalp infection.

◆ Other HIV skin conditions

Drug eruptions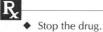

The following drugs are often associated with skin eruptions:

Co-trimoxazole (Bactrim, Septran, Cotrim, Purbac, Ultrazole), amoxycillin, penicillin, INH and dapsone.

Occasionally a Stevens-Johnson reaction (erythema mutiforme) may occur, especially with sulphonamide use.

Treatment

℞

◆ Stop the drug.

◆ Corticosteroids (hydrocortisone or prednisone) can be used in very severe cases.

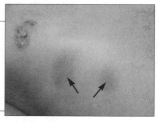

Drug eruption

Urticaria / pruritis / prurigo (itching)

Try to determine the underlying cause and treat this. Folliculitis, scabies, dermatitis and seborrhoeic dermatitis are often responsible for the itching. Dry skin is a common cause.

Treatment

℞

◆ Using bath oils in the bath may be helpful for the dry skin.

◆ Antihistamines e.g. diphenhydramine 50 mg, 6 hourly may relieve symptoms.

◆ Hydroxyzine (Aterax) 25 mg ½ – 1 tablet, 8 – 12 hourly or nightly may also be useful.

(See page 302 for more information on management of dry skin.)

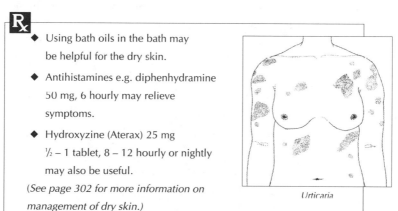

Urticaria

Scabies is a common cause of itching.

Seborrhoeic dermatitis

This usually presents on the scalp, eyebrows, moustache, beard area and upper chest areas. It is very common in immune-deficient patients.

Treatment

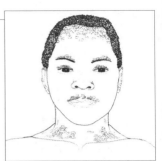

Seborrhoeic dermatitis

℞

- It may be treated with topical steroids, such as 1% hydrocortisone (Betnovate) in UEA. Stronger steroids may be necessary.
- Steroid shampoos and lotions are used for seborrhoeic dermatitis on the scalp and other hairy areas. Selsun shampoo is also useful.
- 2% sulphur in UEA applied nightly can also be used with the steroid cream in more severe cases.
- Liquid paraffin applied first to the scalp lesions may help to loosen the crusts.
- In severe cases, a short-term systemic fungal agent, such as fluconazole is needed.

Psoriasis

Psoriasis is a common HIV-associated condition. It is usually more severe and widespread in HIV-positive people.

Treatment

℞

- Treat with topical steroids, applied locally 12 hourly as above.
- You can also use topical steroids with coal tar preparations e.g. in combination with salicylate ointment.
- Systemic steroids may be needed in severe infection.
- Refer severe cases to a skin specialist.

You may find unusual skin conditions or conditions which do not seem to respond to the usual therapy. You may need to refer to a dermatologist for advice.

Malignancy

Kaposi's sarcoma (KS)

Kaposi's sarcoma may be found anywhere on the skin, in the mouth and palate, or internally in the abdomen, lungs etc. The sarcoma is essentially a tumour of blood capillaries.

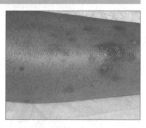

Kaposi's sarcoma on the arm

The lesions usually appear as bluish-black blotches or patches 1 – 2 cm in size. They may grow bigger and other smaller lesions may join to form larger tumours. Skin lesions in themselves do not often cause problems. This tumour is often not painful, however some lesions may cause pain.

KS may appear on the face and other body areas which may cause cosmetic embarrassment. Lesions on the sole of the foot, in the mouth, pharynx or palate may cause discomfort or pressure symptoms. Internal KS may present with a variety of symptoms, depending on which organ is involved.

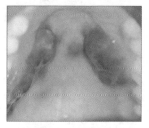

Kaposi's sarcoma on the gums

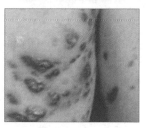

Kaposi's sarcoma on the trunk

Treatment

℞

Treat the lesions if they are cosmetically embarrassing or if they are causing other symptoms.

◆ Lesions of the face or other exposed body parts can be treated locally with intra-lesional therapy using vinblastine or alpha interferon.

◆ Painful lesions or lesions in the mouth, sole of foot or large lesions may be treated with radiotherapy.

◆ Severe, generalised or systemic (internal) KS can be treated with chemotherapy, such as vinblastine, vincristine, bleomycin, adriamycin, VP16 and daunorubicin.

Treatment is often effective. Refer to an oncologist (cancer specialist), dermatologist or radiotherapist for above therapies.

Lymphadenopathy

Swollen lymph nodes are a common finding in HIV disease. Lymphadenopathy is often one of the earliest signs of HIV infection.

The most common cause of lymphadenopathy is the HIV infection itself.

Lymphadenopathy, due to HIV, usually has the following characteristics:

- Lymph glands commonly enlarge in the post-auricular area (behind the ear), in the neck (posteriorly) and in the axilla.

- Enlarged glands may be present in several different areas.

- No local infection is present.

- They usually persist for more than a month.

- Glands are not usually tender or painful.

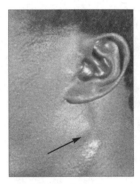

Lymphadenopathy

Look for other causes of lymphadenopathy especially if:

- There is unexplained fever.

- There are very large and/or painful glands.

- Glands are only in one area or unilateral (one-sided).

- There is unexplained weight loss.

- There are other symptoms, such as chronic cough or an enlarged liver or spleen.

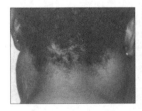

Severe lymphadenopathy

Other important causes of generalised lymphadenopathy in HIV-positive people may need to be considered.

Think of:

- Bacterial infection, such as tuberculosis (large matted nodes, weight loss, cough, night sweats) or secondary syphilis (generalised rashes, fevers)

- Chronic infection with fungi

- Malignancy, such as lymphoma

- Local skin conditions, such as seborrhoeic dermatitis, impetigo, infected lesions

- Sexually transmitted infection, such as syphilis, chancroid, lymphogranuloma venereum (inguinal lymphadenopathy)

You may need to investigate for the most likely causes, depending on other signs and symptoms.

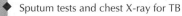

Useful investigatory and diagnostic tests include:

- Full blood count and ESR

- RPR/VDRL non-specific syphilis tests

- Chest X-ray

The following may also be useful:

- Sputum tests and chest X-ray for TB

- PPD skin test for TB

- Viral or fungal serology

- Fine needle aspiration biopsy (FNA) is very useful

- Formal surgical biopsy may be required for diagnosis if FNA is not successful

- A marrow biopsy may be indicated if lymphoma is suspected

Headache

HIV infection can cause headache and dementia (loss of mental functions).

You need to investigate headaches when they have the following characteristics:

◆ Very severe

◆ Not responding to usual simple analgesics

◆ A new and unusual development

◆ Associated with fever

◆ Associated with nausea, vomiting and photophobia

◆ Associated with a fit or faint

◆ Associated with other neurological signs

◆ Associated with signs of meningism (*see the following page*)

If there is a concern about headaches think of:

◆ Meningitis, due to tuberculosis, cryptococcus

◆ Meningo-encephalitis, due to viral infection (e.g. cytomegalovirus)

◆ HIV meningo-encephalitis

◆ Neuro-syphilis

◆ Malignancy, such as lymphoma

◆ Drug side effects, especially if the patient is on zidovudine

◆ Toxoplasmosis of the brain

Remember other usual causes of headache, such as migraine, sinusitis, eye strain, tension (stress), systemic infection (malaria, typhoid, tick bite fever etc.).

Investigations and examinations

- A careful general examination and more specifically a thorough neurological examination must be done to look for:
  - Other signs of meningism (stiff neck, leg raising, high blood pressure, fever)
  - Mental or personality changes e.g. memory loss, confusion
  - Neurological signs of focal brain lesions and raised intracranial pressure, such as cranial nerve palsy and papilloedema. This will be indicated through examination of the retina, abnormal reflexes, abnormal muscle tone, Babinski sign, co-ordination, movement etc.
  - Signs of generalised infection, such as fever, respiratory signs, enlarged liver or spleen, skin rashes, evidence of tuberculosis etc.
- Laboratory investigation may help make a diagnosis, such as a full blood count, blood culture, malaria smear, viral, fungal, rickettsial, toxoplasma, cryptococcal serology and syphilitic tests.
- A lumbar puncture for CSF microscopy, cells and culture may be required for the diagnosis of:
  - Bacterial infection – (neutrophil count)
  - Viral infection – (lymphocyte count)
  - Tuberculosis – (lymphocyte count, electrolytes)
  - Syphilis (RPR / VDRL)
  - Cryptococcal infection (fungi) – india ink microscopic examination
- A brain scan may be required to exclude focal brain lesions, tumour, toxoplasmosis.

Remember to avoid a lumbar puncture if there are signs of raised intracranial pressure with focal signs.

Treatment

Treat the headache with the usual analgesics if symptoms are not severe and if you are confident that you are not dealing with a more serious cause.

In most primary care situations you will need to refer more serious cases to the local hospital or to a consultant physician or neurologist for investigation, treatment or advice.

Cryptococcal meningitis (CM)

Cryptococcal neoformans is a common life-threatening AIDS-related disease. It is acquired from the environment when the fungus is inhaled and multiplies in the lungs. This phase of infection is frequently asymptomatic. The organism can then disseminate widely through the blood stream to skin, bone and the genito-urinary tract, but more commonly to the meninges.

Cryptococcal meningitis usually occurs when the CD4 count is less than 100 cells / mm^3.

Signs and symptoms

◆ Cryptococcal infection is one of the most common causes of meningitis in severe immune-deficient patients (CD4 cell count usually below 75 cells / mm^3).

◆ It is associated with late stage AIDS disease.

◆ The outlook after an infection is very poor.

◆ The onset of CM is usually gradual.

◆ Fever, headache and fatigue are common symptoms.

◆ Neck stiffness may be present and sometimes an altered mental state, confusion, coma and focal neurological signs.

◆ A lumbar puncture will help to diagnose CM. Prior to the lumbar puncture check for papilloedema on retinal inspection.

◆ The diagnosis is confirmed if there is yeast in the cerebro-spinal fluid (CSF), increased CSF pressure, leucocytes (usually lymphocytes), low glucose, increased CSF protein and a positive India ink smear.

◆ A cryptococcal antigen positive result is a valuable test for diagnosing CM. Fungal cultures should be requested if possible.

◆ Untreated, this condition is almost always fatal.

Treatment

℞

◆ Treatment is costly and may not be available in many health care centres.

◆ Refer to hospital for amphotericin 0,7 mg / kg / day for 14 days
  – followed by fluconazole 200 – 400 mg
    daily after meals (indefinitely).
    (see also table on page 156)

Neurological disease

Involvement of the central or peripheral nervous systems is common with HIV and immune-deficiency. Neurological disease is often a feature of advanced immune-deficiency. However some of these conditions may also occur in patients who are not necessarily severely immuno-compromised.

◆ Peripheral neuropathy causes 'pins and needles', and shooting pains or other abnormal sensations around the mouth and in the hands and feet. These are common features of HIV disease.

◆ Peripheral neuropathy may also be due to some commonly used medications such as INH, and many of the ART drugs.

◆ Weakness is another common symptom in people with immune-deficiency.

◆ Focal neurological signs, retinal disease and seizures often indicate infiltration or infection of the central nervous system.

◆ Infection of the meninges is a relatively common opportunistic infection in advanced stages. Unusual forms of meningitis, such as cryptococcal (fungal), syphilitic meningitis or tuberculosis, need to be considered.

◆ Syphilis, tuberculosis and HIV itself are major causes of neurological dysfunction.

◆ Loss of mental function, such as memory, concentration and other cognitive functions, may be part of an overall AIDS-related dementia.

◆ Toxic factors, such as alcohol and drugs (prescription and non-prescription drugs), are occasional causes of neurological signs or symptoms.

Treatment

Rx

- ◆ Referral to specialist centres may be needed for the above conditions.
- ◆ If the patient is under-nourished or has had prolonged diarrhoea, then nutritional deficiencies (Vitamin B, nicotinic acid) should be considered:
    - provide nutritional and vitamin supplements.
- ◆ If dementia or a frank psychosis is present, possible contributing causes should be considered, such as intracranial infection, vitamin deficiencies, alcohol and other possible substance abuse, malaria, etc.
    - referral to a psychiatric institution may be required.
- ◆ Drug therapy may also be a cause of peripheral neuropathy:
    - this must always be considered and the drug discontinued temporarily or permanently;
    - NRTI ARVs such as ddI, 3TC, d4T etc. are known causes of peripheral neuropathy.

Cytomegalovirus (CMV) retinal infection

CMV infections in HIV-positive patients can be very severe. They usually occur in the late stage of the disease when the CD4 levels fall below 50 cells / mm^3. CMV retinitis causes loss of vision and is a cause of blindness. CMV retinitis is diagnosed by finding retinal hemorrhages along the course of ophthalmic vessels and / or yellow-white 'exudates' may surround the patches of bleeding.

Treatment

R$_x$

- ◆ Refer to an ophthalmology unit for advice on therapy.
- ◆ Therapy is usually with ganciclovir or Foscarnet *(see page 156)*.

Toxoplasmosis

Toxoplasmosis is a well-recognised opportunistic infection in patients with severe immune-deficiency (CD4 < 100 cells / mm^3). In healthy people it is usually asymptomatic and is self-limiting.

- ◆ Active toxoplasma disease frequently affects the CNS, the eye (retina), and a variety of other organs especially the lung.

- ◆ It is usually associated with fever and a slow but progressive paralysis (hemiparesis) is characteristic.

- ◆ Toxoplasmosis may be diagnosed in the brain with a CT scan if it is available.

- ◆ Toxoplasmosis of the eye is less common and usually causes a chorio-retinitis. It usually presents with yellow-white, soft spots on the retina. Bleeding is not characteristic of this form of retinitis.

- ◆ Patients who are HIV positive and who present with signs of a fever, stroke or other focal neurological signs should have a thorough assessment to exclude cerebral toxoplasmosis.

- ◆ Diagnosis and treatment should be carried out at a referral centre.

Treatment

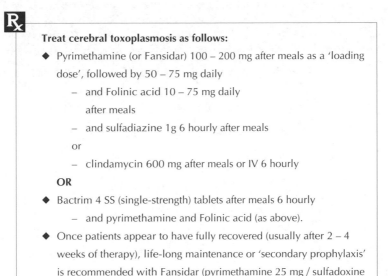

Treat cerebral toxoplasmosis as follows:

◆ Pyrimethamine (or Fansidar) 100 – 200 mg after meals as a 'loading dose', followed by 50 – 75 mg daily

 – and Folinic acid 10 – 75 mg daily
 after meals

 – and sulfadiazine 1g 6 hourly after meals

 or

 – clindamycin 600 mg after meals or IV 6 hourly

OR

◆ Bactrim 4 SS (single-strength) tablets after meals 6 hourly

 – and pyrimethamine and Folinic acid (as above).

◆ Once patients appear to have fully recovered (usually after 2 – 4 weeks of therapy), life-long maintenance or 'secondary prophylaxis' is recommended with Fansidar (pyrimethamine 25 mg / sulfadoxine 500 mg = 1 tablet twice weekly).

See also page 156.

Fever (pyrexia)

Fever of 38ºC or higher which lasts more than 2 weeks (and is the only clinical sign) may occur in an HIV-positive person.

HIV infection itself can cause a low grade fever (37º – 38ºC). When fever is higher, and lasts for an ongoing period, then you will need to look for other causes.

Ongoing fever without any other clinical signs or symptoms should make you think of:

◆ *Mycobacterium tuberculosis* or other unusual mycobacterium infections e.g. *Mycobacterium avium*

◆ Systemic fungal infection, especially cryptococcus

◆ Bacterial infection due to

 – salmonella   – *Haemophilus influenzae*

 – *Streptococcus pneumoniae*   – syphilis

◆ Viral infections, especially cytomegalovirus (CMV)

◆ Protozoal infection, especially

 – *Pneumocystis carinii*   – *Toxoplasma gondii*

◆ Malignancy e.g. lymphoma

**Common causes of unexplained fever
in advanced HIV infection are tuberculosis or *Pneumocystis carinii* infection.
Occasionally the HIV infection itself may cause the fever.**

Investigations and examinations (fever)

Try to determine the cause for the ongoing fever.

The folowing investigations may be helpful:

◆ Full blood count

◆ RPR/VDRL

◆ Sputum for acid fast bacilli

◆ Blood, urine and stool culture

◆ Serology for toxoplasma, CMV virus and cryptococcus

◆ Chest X-ray

**If these tests do not help diagnose the cause, you may need to refer the
patient to hospital for:**

◆ Lumbar puncture, especially looking for meningitis
  e.g. cryptococcal meningitis (an india ink microscopy),
  tuberculosis, viral meningo-encephalitis

◆ A bone marrow biospsy, looking for tuberculosis, lymphoma and
  bacterial infection

◆ Bronchoscopy, for *Pneumocystis carinii*

◆ Ultrasound may help detect a malignant tumour
  e.g. an intra-abdominal lymphoma

◆ Brain scan, for toxoplasma and tumour

Treatment

R̲x

**Therapy is otherwise determined by the results of the above tests
and the cause. If you are unable to find the cause then consider
the following:**

◆ In the primary care setting, you could consider giving a 10 – 14 day
  course of a broad-spectrum antibiotic treatment.
  Co-trimoxazole plus ampicillin/amoxycillin or chloramphenicol
  are useful antibiotics to try, as they cover common bacterial
  infections and an early *Pneumocystis carinii* pneumonia infection.

◆ Refer to a specialist centre for assistance.

Weight loss

Weight loss is common and may be due to the HIV infection in itself or due to an HIV-related infection or malignancy.

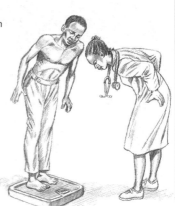

The following are more common causes of weight loss:

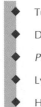

- Tuberculosis
- Diarrhoea
- *Pneumocystis carinii*
- Lymphoma
- HIV infection itself

Try to find and treat the cause of the weight loss.

Investigate for the above causes. Often you will not be able to find the cause as it is frequently due to the HIV infection itself.

Treatment

℞ Manage with high calorie and protein diet such as:

- ◆ Frequent small meals with high-energy foods, such as porridge, potato, rice
- ◆ High protein foods, such as eggs, milk, beans, lentils, meat, fish
- ◆ Commercial high-energy and calorie preparations, such as PVM, Complan and Ensure are useful, if available

Weight loss is usually a sign of an underlying opportunistic infection or a sign of advanced HIV infection.

Treatment and secondary prophylaxis of opportunistic infections in adults

Standard adult doses have been given. Every effort has been made to check doses, but readers should check other sources. Usual duration of therapy has been given, but longer courses may be needed in individual cases.

Infection	Treatment options	Duration	Secondary prophylaxis[1]
Herpes simplex	Valciclovir 500 mg 2 x daily Acyclovir 400 mg 3 x daily Famciclovir 125 mg 2 x daily	7 days	Not usually recommended (acyclovir 400 mg 2 x daily)
Tuberculosis	Standard short-course therapy	6 months	Not recommended
Candida oesophagitis	Fluconazole 100 mg daily Itraconazole 200 mg daily Ketoconazole 400 mg daily	14 – 28 days	Not recommended

Infection	Treatment options	Duration	Secondary prophylaxis[1]
Pneumocystis carinii pneumonia[2]	Co-trimoxazole[3] 3 – 4 tabs 4 x daily Dapsone 100 mg daily **plus** trimethoprim 300 mg 3 x daily Clindamycin 450 mg 3 x daily **plus** primaquine 15 mg daily	14 – 21 days	Co-trimoxazole[3] 2 tabs daily Dapsone 100 mg daily
Toxoplasmosis	Co-trimoxazole[3] 4 tabs 2 x daily **then** 2 tabs 2 x daily Clindamycin 600 mg 4 x daily **plus** pyrimethamine[4] 50 mg daily	4 weeks 12 weeks 6 weeks	Co-trimoxazole[3] 2 tabs daily
Cytomegalovirus	Ganciclovir 5 mg / kg 2 x daily IV **then** Ganciclovir 5 mg / kg / day IV 5 days / week or 1 g 3 x daily orally	14 days Lifelong[1]	N/A
Atypical mycobacteriosis	Clarithromycin 500 mg 2 x daily **plus** ethambutol 800 mg daily	Lifelong[1]	N/A
Salmonella bacteraemia Isosporiasis	Ciprofloxacin 500 mg 2 x daily Co-trimoxazole[3] 4 tabs 2x daily Pyrimethamine[4] 25 mg daily	6 weeks 4 weeks	Not recommended Co-trimoxazole[3] 2 tabs daily Pyrimethamine[4] 75 mg daily
Cryptosporidiosis	N/A (anti-motility drugs)	N/A	N/A
Bacterial pneumonia	Cefuroxime 750 mg – 1,5 g 3 x daily IV[5] Cefamandole 1 – 2 g 4 x daily IV[5] Ceftriaxone 1 – 2 g daily IV[5] Cefotaxime 1 – 2 g 2 x daily IV[5] Co-amoxiclav 1.2 g 3 x daily IV[5] Moxifloxacin 400 mg daily Gatifloxacin 400 mg daily	5 – 10 days	Not recommended
Cryptococcal meningitis	Amphotericin B 0,7 mg / kg[6] IV daily **then** fluconazole 400 mg daily	7 – 14 days 8 – 10 weeks	Fluconazole 100 – 200 mg daily[4]
Herpes zoster (shingles)	Acyclovir 800 mg 5 times / day Valaciclovir 1 g 3 x daily Famciclovir 250 mg 3 x daily	7 days	Not recommended
Microsporidiosis	Albendazole 400 mg 2 x daily[7]	21 days	Not recommended

1. Prophylaxis or lifelong therapy can be discontinued if the CD4 count increases to > 200 on ART.

2. Adjunctive corticosteroids are indicated in hypoxic patients (oral prednisone 40 mg 2 x daily followed by a steady reduction after 5 – 10 days).

3. Single-strength (480 mg) tablets.

4. Folinic acid (not folic acid) should be used to treat or prevent bone marrow suppression.

5. Therapy should be completed with oral antibiotics (amoxicillin, co-amoxiclav, moxifloxacin or gatifloxacin are recommended). These antibiotics are recommended in the South African Thoracic Society guidelines on community-acquired pneumonia (in press).

6. A test dose of 1 mg should be given over 30 minutes. If this is tolerated, then half the daily dose can be infused over 4 hours with the full dose given the next day. Many experts omit the test dose.

7. Only certain species (notably *Encephalitozoon intestinalis*) respond well to albendazole.

Source: 'The prevention and treatment of opportunistic infections in HIV infected adults'
The Southern African Journal of HIV Medicine, March 2002, 7, pages 17 – 20

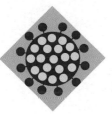

Chapter 8

CHILDREN WITH HIV INFECTION AND AIDS

HIV infection in newborn babies and children

The diagnosis of HIV infection in newborn babies and children

Common HIV-associated conditions in children

Clinical categories for children with HIV infection

Management of children with HIV infection

Anti-retroviral therapy (ART) for children

Recognising and treating HIV-associated infections and conditions

Preventing opportunistic infections

Hospitalisation of children with HIV/AIDS

Counselling and support

Immunisation of children with HIV infection

HIV infection in newborn babies and children

◆ The AIDS epidemic in children

As the HIV epidemic increases many more children become infected with HIV. `

The onset of AIDS in children is usually much earlier than in an adult. A significant proportion of HIV-infected children will develop AIDS and die within the first 2 years of life. Many of the child health care units are experiencing large numbers of admissions due to AIDS because the epidemic in children peaks earlier than in adults.

The quality of such care will vary depending on:

- the skills of the individual health care worker
- the type of care that is provided
- the resources available at any particular time

It is well recognised that resources for health care differ widely. HIV care can be costly, and some of the care recommendations may not be affordable in some health services. Hopefully drug prices may reduce in the future and additional care options may become possible. This guide will attempt to be as realistic as possible, but at times may suggest care options which may not always be affordable by all.

In all areas there needs to be good, ongoing communication for discussion and referral between primary, secondary or tertiary child care facilities for HIV/AIDS. Health care workers also need to be aware of community-based structures within their regions which can provide care and support for HIV-infected children and their families.

◆ HIV viral patterns in babies and children

HIV viral activity in children is different from that seen in adults. In adults, high viral levels occur in the first weeks after infection and reach a steady state approximately 4 – 6 months after the primary HIV infection *(see page 76)*. The steady state is due to the immune response, which helps to prevent HIV viral replication. The level of HIV (viral load) in the steady state can help to predict the disease progression and overall future outcome (prognosis).

In babies, there is a very rapid increase in HIV viral levels in the first weeks of life in perinatally acquired HIV infection (10 000 – 10 000 000). These levels remain very high for the first 1 – 2 years of life (not 4 – 6 months as in adults). They gradually decline over the next few years, reaching a 'steady state' by the age of about 5 – 6 years.

Viral load in relation to early or late infection in children

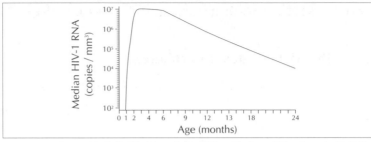

Source: Martin D. 'Viral dynamics in children.' Southern African Journal of HIV Medicine, October 2002, page 12

◆ Most children acquire HIV infection during pregnancy, childbirth and breast feeding

Children usually acquire HIV infection from their mothers during pregnancy, childbirth and breast feeding. Approximately 25 – 30% of HIV-positive mothers will transmit HIV to their babies, a significant proportion of infection being transmitted through breast milk. There is a risk of infection from breast feeding during the entire period of feeding. The longer the period of breast feeding the higher the risk. This risk probably increases when complementary foods are added to breast milk, which is why exclusive breast feeding is recommended for up to 6 months.

Some children have also become infected from blood transfusions and from being sexually abused.

On average, about 60% of transmitted infection is transmitted during childbirth, 10 – 20% during pregnancy and 20 – 40% during breast feeding.

A mother seems more likely to pass on the virus to her foetus during pregnancy, childbirth or breast feeding if:

◆ She becomes HIV-infected just before the pregnancy or during the pregnancy.

◆ She has advanced (symptomatic) HIV disease with:
   – a high HIV viral load (< 100 000)
   – a low CD4 cell count
   – symptoms of AIDS

◆ If the mother has a low viral load (< 1 000), HIV transmission is unlikely.

> **There is a 25 – 30% chance that an HIV-positive mother will pass on the virus to her unborn foetus during pregnancy, childbirth or breast feeding. Most of these infections can be prevented.**
> *MTCT and ways to prevent it are discussed in Chapter 10.*

◆ Development of symptoms

The clinical course of HIV infection differs significantly in children compared with adults.

- ◆ The time from infection to the development of AIDS, and finally to death, is generally much shorter in children than in adults.

- ◆ A larger proportion of children will develop serious illness and death within the first year or two of life.

- ◆ It is estimated that 75% of all HIV-infected children will have died before their fifth birthday (without ART).

Children, as in adults, can be divided into two main groups – rapid and slow progressors.

Rapid progressors

- ◆ These children are usually symptomatic by 6 – 12 months of age.

- ◆ They develop more severe illnesses and die within the first 2 years of life.

- ◆ About 40 – 60% of children with HIV are rapid progressors.

Rapidly progressing children usually have:

- ◆ High viral loads

- ◆ Low CD4 cell counts *(see table on page 174)*

The progress to AIDS may be accelerated by:

- ◆ Poor nutritional state

- ◆ Illnesses such as TB, malaria, measles, respiratory infections, gastro-enteritis

Slow progressors

- ◆ These children develop symptoms some time after the first year of life.

- ◆ They have a milder illness and a longer survival period (2 – 7 years).

- ◆ Some may survive to older childhood, and even into the early teenage years.

- ◆ In Africa, HIV-infected children who do not get ART usually do not survive past the age of 5 years.

The diagnosis of HIV infection in newborn babies and children

CHILDREN WITH HIV/AIDS

The foetus may passively acquire HIV antibodies from the mother during pregnancy

If a mother is HIV-infected, she can pass on her HIV **antibodies** to her foetus during pregnancy. These **antibodies** will show up on an HIV ELISA antibody test. By 18 months (usually 12 – 15 months) the mother's antibodies (in the foetus) will have disappeared.

This means that a newborn can test HIV antibody positive for up to 18 months of life, without being truly HIV-infected. In other words, the baby has just passively acquired the antibodies from the mother and has not acquired the HIV virus.

It is possible to do a PCR HIV test on the baby *(see page 46)*. This tests for evidence of the HIV virus. A PCR test can determine whether an HIV antibody positive baby is truly infected. PCR tests are more reliable 28 days or more after birth.

> **A positive HIV antibody test in the first 12 – 15 months of life is an unreliable test, and does not necessarily mean that the child has HIV infection.**

◆ The diagnosis of AIDS in a newborn should include the following:

An HIV positive antibody or PCR test in the baby or mother

This means that either the baby or the mother will be found to be HIV positive.

It should also include at least three of the following:

- ◆ Failure to thrive or weight loss
- ◆ Prolonged fever
- ◆ Recurrent oral thrush
- ◆ Persistent generalised lymphadenopathy
- ◆ Lymphoid interstitial pneumonitis
- ◆ Chronic diarrhoea
- ◆ Tuberculosis (pulmonary or extra-pulmonary)
- ◆ Recurrent bacterial infection
- ◆ Opportunistic infections *(see page 166)*
- ◆ Encephalopathy *(see page 166)*

Advanced HIV infection would also include laboratory findings that may show any of the following:

- Low haemoglobin, neutrophils and platelets

- Low CD4 (T4) cell count (absolute count or a low percentage < 15%)
  See page 174

- High HIV viral load

- Abnormally elevated gamma-globulin levels (they may also be reduced)

Remember that it is often difficult to diagnose HIV infection in a child under 18 months. A positive HIV antibody test alone may not indicate actual HIV infection. If you suspect that the child has HIV, you should check the child's progress every 3 – 6 months, and repeat the HIV antibody test at around 18 months of age (to allow any maternal HIV antibodies to disappear).

However, if the child becomes ill, especially with the conditions listed above, then HIV infection is more likely. An HIV PCR test (*see the following page and Chapter 4*) can detect HIV infection within the first month of life and becomes reliable after about 4 weeks of life.

◆ World Health Organisation (WHO) paediatric classification of HIV/AIDS

Stage I

- ◆ Asymptomatic

- ◆ Generalised lymphadenopathy

Stage II

- ◆ Unexplained chronic diarrhoea

- ◆ Recurrent severe bacterial infection

- ◆ Oral candidiasis beyond neonatal period (severe, persistent or recurrent)

- ◆ Persistent fever

Stage III

- ◆ AIDS opportunistic infections (TB, cryptococcal meningitis, PCP etc.)

- ◆ Severe failure to thrive

- ◆ Progressive encephalopathy

- ◆ Recurrent septicaemia

- ◆ Malignancy

◆ HIV tests for children

HIV PCR RNA test

More sophisticated tests can be done to check for the presence of the HIV virus in a newborn within the first few months of life e.g.

- – an HIV RNA polymerase chain reaction (PCR)

However, these are often too expensive and too sophisticated for general use, and are not usually available outside the major cities. The HIV PCR test becomes reliable approximately 1 month after the baby's birth.

Diagnosis of HIV infection often relies on the child's clinical condition

The clinical condition of a child, in the first 2 years of life, is usually a good way to know if a child is infected or not.

- ◆ A child whose mother is HIV positive, and who is very sickly in the first year of life, is likely to be HIV-infected.

- ◆ A child who is thriving and who remains well in the first 2 years of life, is most likely free from HIV infection, or is one of the slower progressors.

Positive HIV antibody test

An HIV antibody test which is positive **after the first year of life** is suggestive of HIV infection, and if it is positive **after 18 months** the child is almost certainly HIV-infected.

On the other hand, a baby who is HIV positive after birth, and later becomes HIV negative, is most likely to be free of HIV infection.

In a newborn baby of an HIV-positive mother, the ELISA test could be repeated at 3 – 6 monthly intervals until the age of 18 months. However, if the child is doing well and thriving, it is often only necessary to re-test the child at the 15 – 18 month period. A child who has not been actually infected with HIV will have a negative ELISA HIV antibody test by 15 – 18 months of age.

The usual ethical and legal obligations must be carried out when testing babies and children for HIV.

Ethical considerations when doing HIV tests on babies and children

◆ Informed consent from the parent or legal guardian is necessary

   – the superintendent of the hospital can sign consent in
      urgent situations if the parent or guardian is unavailable.

◆ The necessary pre- and post-test counselling for the parent / guardian, or for an older child, must be provided. Explain the following to families, as part of the pre-test counselling:

   – routine antibody test results reflect the mother's
      HIV status, not necessarily that of the baby;

   – if definitive antigen or PCR tests are not available,
      there may be a waiting period until the diagnosis
      can be established;

   – it may be necessary to repeat the tests and
      wait until the child is 15 – 18 months of
      age or older before the diagnosis is
      finally confirmed (if a PCR test is
      not possible).

*The clinical condition of a child, in the first 2 years
of life, is usually a good way to know if a child is infected or not.*

> **Children over the age of 18 months, who are HIV positive, are likely to be truly HIV positive and must be regarded as being HIV-infected.**

Common HIV-associated conditions in children

Children with HIV infection often present with non-specific conditions which are commonly found in general paediatrics.

◆ The most commonly associated conditions

   ◆ Failure to gain weight (failure to thrive) or malnutrition
   ◆ Persistent and generalised lymphadenopathy and / or enlarged liver and spleen
   ◆ Recurrent or ongoing diarrhoeal disease
   ◆ Dermatitis and seborrhoeic dermatitis
   ◆ Oral thrush (candidiasis)

◆ Prolonged fever

◆ Anaemia and thrombocytopaenia platelet deficiency

◆ Severe and recurring bacterial infections. Organisms commonly causing infections include pneumococci, streptococci, staphylococci, *Haemophilus influenzae* and salmonella.

These infections may cause:

- upper respiratory tract infection, including otitis media
- pneumonia
- skin infection, such as cellulitis, abscesses, impetigo
- urinary tract infection
- meningitis
- osteomyelitis

◆ Swelling of the parotid salivary gland

◆ Tuberculosis of the lung and / or other organs

◆ Lymphoid interstitial pneumonitis (LIP)

◆ Opportunistic infections are a sign of late-stage HIV infection and may include:

- repeated oral thrush (candidiasis)
- tuberculosis
- *Pneumocystis carinii* pneumonia
- disseminated viral infection, especially with herpes or cytomegalovirus
- toxoplasmosis

◆ Neurological damage by HIV infection may result in encephelopathy, especially in advanced HIV infection.

◆ Signs of encephalopathy include:

- developmental delay or regression of milestones already reached
- seizures (fits)
- reduced head growth / size (microcephaly)
- other abnormal neurological findings

(see diagram on page 173)

◆ The most common clinical syndromes

Wasting syndrome

◆ Failure to thrive is often associated with wasting (best seen on the thighs) and / or chronic or recurrent diarrhoeal disease.

◆ It may be due to:

- the direct effect of HIV infection on the gastro-intestinal tract, secondary opportunistic infections (such as cryptosporidium, cytomegalovirus and other viruses and bacteria)
- poor nutritional intake

Persistent generalised lymphadenopathy

◆ This may be with or without hepatosplenomegaly and parotid enlargement.

Recurrent bacterial infections

◆ These are of varying severity and include septicaemia, meningitis, pneumonia, otitis media, tonsillitis, cellulitis and urinary tract infections.

Respiratory diseases

◆ Bacterial pneumonia, recurrent chest infections, tuberculosis.

◆ *Pneumocystis carinii* pneumonia (PCP) is characterised by sudden onset of fever, tachypnoea, hypoxaemia and a diffuse interstitial infiltrate on X-ray. It occurs most commonly in children under one and is usually associated with a very poor prognosis.

Lymphoid interstitial pneumonia (LIP)

◆ This is a slowly progressive interstitial lung disease of unknown cause.

◆ It is characterised by bilateral reticulonodular infiltrates and mediastinal lymphadenopathy on chest X-ray.

◆ LIP is commonly associated with parotomegaly and clubbing.

◆ It is often asymptomatic and usually has a good prognosis.

Tuberculosis

◆ The manifestations of tuberculosis are usually no different to non-HIV infected persons, except that the disease may be atypical or severe in children with immune-deficiency.

◆ Diagnosis of TB in children is often difficult and made on clinical suspicion.

◆ The TB may also be pulmonary or extra-pulmonary and frequently in the lymph nodes.

Neurological syndromes

◆ These conditions may be due to a variety of reasons.

◆ Progressive encephalopathy may manifest as developmental delay or loss of developmental milestones, convulsions or behavioural abnormalities.

Dermatitis

◆ Skin rashes are common. These include severe nappy rash and allergic skin eruptions.

◆ Extensive seborrhoeic dermatitis is common.

Opportunistic, HIV-related infections

◆ These often include:
- tuberculosis
- *Pneumocystis carinii*
- candida (thrush)
- cytomegalovirus, cryptosporidium, mycobacterium tuberculosis
- herpes simplex

Blood disorders

◆ These include anaemia, neutropaenia and thrombocytopaenia.

◆ They present with pallor, infections or bleeding (especially nose bleeds).

◆ Nutritional deficiencies (iron and folate) can make the anaemia worse.

Young children (under 1 year) tend to present with symptoms such as failure to thrive, acute or recurrent diarrhoeal disease, severe sepsis and PCP. The severe nature of these conditions is reflected in the poor prognosis of children who present at this age. Children over 1 year of age tend to present with milder disease such as hepatosplenomegaly, lymphadenopathy, parotitis and recurrent bacterial infections.

Clinical categories for children with HIV infection

Category N: not symptomatic

Children who have no signs or symptoms considered to be the result of HIV infection or who have only one of the conditions listed in Category A.

Category A: mildly symptomatic

Children with two or more of the conditions listed below, but none of the conditions listed in Categories B and C.

◆ Lymphadenopathy (> 0,5 cm at more than two sites; bilateral = one site)

◆ Hepatomegaly

◆ Splenomegaly

◆ Dermatitis

◆ Parotitis

◆ Recurrent or persistent upper respiratory infection, sinusitis or otitis media

Category B: moderately symptomatic

Children who have symptomatic conditions other than those listed in Categories A or C that are attributed to HIV infection. Examples of conditions in clinical Category B include, but are not limited to:

◆ Anaemia (< 8 gm / dL), neutropaenia (< 1 000 / mm^3) or thrombocytopaenia (< 100 000 / mm^3) persisting > 30 days

◆ Bacterial meningitis, pneumonia or sepsis (single episode)

◆ Candidiasis, oropharyngeal (thrush), persisting > 2 months in children > 6 months of age

◆ Cardiomyopathy

◆ Cytomegalovirus infection, with onset before 1 month of age

◆ Diarrhoea, recurrent or chronic

◆ Hepatitis

◆ Herpes simplex virus (HSV), stomatitis, recurrent (more than two episodes within 1 year)

◆ Hepatitis

◆ Herpes simplex virus (HSV), stomatitis, recurrent (more than two episodes within 1 year)

◆ HSV bronchitis, pneumonitis or oesophagitis with onset before 1 month of age

◆ Herpes zoster (shingles) involving at least two distinct episodes or more than one dermatome

◆ Leiomyosarcoma

◆ Lymphoid interstitial pneumonia (LIP) or pulmonary lymphoid hyperplasia complex

◆ Nephropathy

◆ Nocardiosis

◆ Persistent fever (lasting > 1 month)

◆ Toxoplasmosis, onset before 1 month of age

◆ Varicella, disseminated (complicated chickenpox)

Category C: severely symptomatic

Serious bacterial infections, multiple or recurrent i.e. any combination of at least two culture-confirmed infections within a 3-year period) of the following types:

- septicaemia

- pneumonia

- meningitis

- bone or joint infection

- abscess of an internal organ or body cavity
  (excluding otitis media, superficial skin or mucosal abscesses)

- indwelling catheter-related infections

◆ Candidiasis, oesophageal or pulmonary (bronchi, trachea, lungs)

◆ Coccidioidomycosis, disseminated (at site other than, or in addition to, lungs, or cervical or hilar lymph nodes)

◆ Cryptococcosis, extrapulmonary

◆ Cryptosporidiosis or isosporiasis with diarrhoea persisting > 1 month

◆ Cytomegalovirus disease with onset of symptoms at age > 1 month (at a site other than liver, spleen or lymph nodes)

◆ Encephalopathy with at least one of the following progressive findings present for at least 2 months, in the absence of a concurrent illness other than HIV infection that could explain the findings:

- failure to attain or loss of developmental milestones
  or loss of intellectual ability, verified by standard
  developmental scale or neuropsychological tests

- impaired brain growth or acquired microcephaly
  demonstrated by head circumference measurements
  or brain atrophy demonstrated by computerised
  tomography or magnetic resonance imaging (serial
  imaging is required for children < 2 years of age)

- acquired symmetric motor deficit manifested by two
  or more of the following: paresis, pathologic reflexes,
  ataxia or gait disturbance

◆ Herpes simplex virus infection causing a mucocutaneous ulcer that persists for > 1 month

- **or** bronchitis, pneumonitis or oesophagitis for any
  duration affecting a child > 1 month of age

Category C (continued)

◆ Histoplasmosis, disseminated (at a site other than, or in addition to, lungs, or cervical or hilar lymph nodes)

◆ Kaposi's sarcoma

◆ Lymphoma, primary, in brain

  – **or** small, non-cleaved cell (Burkitt's)
  – **or** immunoblastic
  – **or** large cell lymphoma
  – **or** B-cell
  – **or** unknown immunologic phenotype

◆ Mycobacterium tuberculosis, disseminated or extrapulmonary

◆ Mycobacterium, other species or unidentified species, disseminated (at a site other than, or in addition to, lungs, skin, or cervical or hilar lymph nodes)

◆ *Mycobacterium avium* complex or *Mycobacterium kansasii*, disseminated (at site other than, or in addition to, lungs, skin, or cervical or hilar lymph nodes)

◆ *Pneumocystis carinii* pneumonia

◆ Progressive multifocal leukoencephalopathy

◆ Salmonella (non-typhoid) septicaemia, recurrent

◆ Toxoplasmosis of the brain with onset at > 1 month of age

◆ Wasting syndrome in the absence of a concurrent illness other than HIV infection that could explain the following findings:

  – persistent weight loss > 10% of baseline

  – **or** downward crossing of at least two of the following percentile lines on the weight-for-age chart (e.g. 95th, 75th, 50th, 25th, 5th) in a child > 1 year of age

  – **or** < 5th percentile on weight-for-height chart on two consecutive measurements, ≥ 30 days apart **plus** chronic diarrhoea (i.e. ≥ loose stools per day for ≥ 30 days)

  – **or** documented fever (for ≥ 30 days, intermittent or constant)

Management of children with HIV infection

Management aims to keep the child well and symptom-free for as long as possible. Try to keep the child at home and out of hospital as much as possible.

> **Management of children with HIV infection includes:**
>
> ◆ Regular medical and growth checks
>
> ◆ ART
>
> ◆ Recognising and aggressively treating infections and abnormal conditions
>
> ◆ Preventing opportunistic infections
>
> ◆ Nutritional care and support
>
> ◆ Counselling and general supportive care

Remember to ensure that the child is fully immunised.

◆ Regular medical and growth checks

Check the child at regular intervals i.e. every 2 – 3 months, or more frequently if the child is ill.

Keep a close watch on the following:

◆ Developmental progress and monitoring of growth

◆ Weight gain or loss (regular growth charting)

◆ Head size

◆ Adequate nourishment and feeding – you may need to supply nutritional supplements, such as milk, and / or protein, vitamin and mineral (PVM) mixtures, especially if the child is bottle fed, underweight or malnourished.

Take a careful history

Ask the parent / guardian about the following:

◆ History of the pregnancy, immunisation, previous illness and social circumstances

◆ Fever

◆ Poor feeding, failure to gain weight or to develop normally

◆ Coughs, diarrhoea, skin rashes, swellings, thrush

◆ Shortness of breath

◆ Any other new problems

◆ Any symptoms of any of the conditions outlined *on the following page*

General examination

Do a general examination looking for any new clinical developments.

Keep a special look-out for the HIV-related conditions shown below:

Common HIV-associated conditions in young children *(see also page 165)*

Neurological conditions

Reduced head size
Poor general tone
Poor developmental progress
Encephalopathy
Meningitis

Upper respiratory tract conditions

Oral diseases, especially candida (thrush)
Signs of malnutrition
Otitis media
Tonsillitis
Pharyngitis

Lower respiratory tract conditions

Acute pneumonias
Tuberculosis
Pneumocystis carinii
LIP (Lymphoid interstitial pneumonia)

Wasting

Signs of wasting and
nutritional deficiency

General problems

Weight loss
(road to health chart)
Malnutrition
Pallor (anaemia)
Fever/pyrexia

Parotid gland
Enlarged

Lymph nodes

Swellings of the
lymph nodes
in the neck,
axilla and
groin

Skin conditions

Skin diseases e.g.
Herpes zoster
herpes simplex
dermatitis/eczema
bacterial infections

Liver / spleen
An enlarged liver or spleen

Failure to thrive or weight loss is worrying in a child with HIV infection and may be the first sign of an underlying opportunistic infection or development of AIDS.

◆ Laboratory tests

General assessment

 Do a full blood count and platelet count.

Tests to assess immune function

◆ Total lymphocyte count (reduced in immune-deficiency)

◆ CD4 (T4) lymphocyte count and percentage *(see below)*

Laboratory monitoring

The CD4 count is an important marker of the immune status. Ideally CD4 cells should be monitored at least every 3 – 4 months if affordable. The table below outlines the expected CD4 cell counts according to the age of the child and the severity of immune-deficiency.

Immune status	Age of child					
	< 12 months		1 – 5 years		6 – 12 years	
Immunologic category	CD4 / mm³	%	CD4 / mm³	%	CD4 / mm³	%
◆ No immuno-suppression (normal)	≥ 1500	≥ 25	≥ 1 000	≥ 25	≥ 500	≥ 25
◆ Moderate immuno-supression	750 – 1 499	15 – 24	500 – 999	15 – 24	200 – 499	15 – 24
◆ Severe immuno-suppression	< 750	< 15	< 500	< 15	< 200	< 15

◆ **The HIV PCR viral load** test is not yet widely available, but is very important in assessing:
   – whether an HIV-positive baby is truly infected with HIV *(see page 162)*
   – the severity of the infection
   – the effect of anti-retroviral therapy (ART)

◆ Also **immunoglobulin levels** (usually elevated gamma-globulin in HIV infection) can be checked.

◆ Investigations should initially be done on diagnosis (as a baseline) and 3 – 6 months thereafter depending on resources. They should be done more frequently if the child's clinical condition warrants it.

Other tests

◆ Chest X-ray, especially if there are signs suggestive of respiratory distress, tuberculosis, failure to thrive or weight loss.

◆ Investigation of a fever or infection, with throat swabs, urine, stool or blood cultures etc., may also be needed.

◆ Investigation of other abnormal clinical findings or laboratory tests must be carried out as usual.

Anti-retroviral therapy (ART) for children

ART is a rapidly developing option for the treatment of children with HIV. Consultation with experienced paediatricians is advised. A number of effective ARV drugs are now available. However the cost of the drugs limit their general usage. Where resources permit, ART should be initiated in HIV-infected patients at an appropriate stage in their clinical course. In general, ART in children follows the same principles as in adult therapy. It should be remembered that HIV viral loads are higher in the first year of life, and reduce and settle only after approximately 5 – 6 years *(see page 159)*. Viral levels are usually very high in the first 2 years, often ranging from 100 000 – 10 000 000 RNA copies / mm^3 (averaging approximately 185 000 copies / mm^3). A combination of viral load and CD4 cell count is a good predictor of future outcome.

The aims of ART in children are:

◆ Preservation or restoration of immune function (CD4 cell count)

◆ Maximum and ongoing suppression of viral load

◆ Improvement in and maintenance of health status

◆ Reduction in ill health and death

In general, ART should result in improved quality of life in the child, and promote wellness as well as social, physical and intellectual development. Reducing illness and hospitalisation will be hugely beneficial to the child's health and also to the health and welfare of the family.

The two clinical situations when ART should be considered are when:

◆ There is early diagnosis of HIV infection. This is when HIV infection is confirmed in a baby less than 3 months of age (whose mother is HIV positive) by a positive HIV PCR test and a viral load assessment.

◆ A child or baby is diagnosed late due to:
    – the development of HIV-related symptomatic disease or
    – because of a positive HIV diagnosis in the mother.

◆ Combination therapy

Ideally, 3 drugs should be used (if there is a very high viral load a fourth drug may be added). This will help in suppressing viral replication and preventing the development of drug resistance. There may be a role for dual (2-drug) therapy in children with less advanced disease, where cost or adherence to therapy is a problem.

◆ Good adherence

Good adherence to therapy is critical to the achievement of a satisfactory viral and immunological outcome. Adequate adherence is affected by:

- The motivation and commitment of the caregiver and family support
- The patient's ability to pay for the drugs on an ongoing basis if they are not provided by the health care services
- The caregiver's understanding of the importance of adherence and of the correct drug regimen
- Access to regular follow-up care and support

For successful ART, at least 80% adherence to drug therapy is usually required.

◆ When to start ART

In children, ART should be started once one of the two following events occur:

- Clinical Category B is reached *(see table on page 169)*. (If Category B is only due to a single episode of a bacterial infection or herpes zoster, then wait until Category C is reached.)
- Clinical Category C is reached.
- Children need ART if they are:
  - very ill
  - getting repeated opportunistic infections
  - losing weight / not thriving
- There is a CD4 cell percentage of less than 20% *(see table on page 174).*

◆ Monitoring children on ART

The CD4 cell count and percentage

The CD4 cell count is very important:

- in assessing the stage of the disease
- in assessing when to start therapy
- for monitoring the effect of therapy.

Actual CD4 counts are higher in children than adults. It is often more useful to monitor the CD4 percentage (i.e. the percentage of CD4 cells over the CD3 lymphocyte or over the total lymphocyte count). *Values for CD4 cells are provided in the table on page 174.*

General points to remember:

◆ A persistent drop in CD4 count or percentage together with evidence of clinical deterioration (loss of weight, failure to thrive, appearance of oral thrush and other infections) is evidence of ART failure.

◆ In children, a CD4 cell percentage below 15% indicates advanced immune-deficiency, and is comparative to a CD4 cell count below 200 cells / mm³ in an adult.

◆ There is a high likelihood of opportunistic infections when the CD4 cells reach low levels (< 15 – 20%), although some infections (e.g. PCP pneumonia) may occur even if the CD4 cell counts are within 'normal' ranges.

◆ CD4 cell measures should ideally be done every 4 – 6 months if affordable.

◆ A rising or stable CD4 cell count or percentage (after it was steadily dropping) is an indication of successful ART. A falling CD4 count or percentage means the ART is failing.

◆ CD4 counts can be temporarily lowered for a month or more if there is an infection in the child or if a vaccination has been given.

◆ Repeat any test with an unexpected CD4 cell count result.

◆ Two measurements 1 month apart should be done before making any significant clinical care change if the change is based on the CD4 count.

> **The CD4 cell count is the most important indicator of the health status of a child (and adult) with HIV infection. The health status is usually good if the CD4 cell count is in a favourable situation (improved / stable after it was steadily declining). In a child, a CD4 cell percentage below 15% indicates advanced immune-deficiency. It has similar meaning to a CD4 cell count below 200 cells / mm³ in an adult.**

The HIV viral load

The viral load should also be monitored if possible. This can be done with the CD4 cell count monitoring.

◆ Viral loads may temporarily rise for up to a month after infections or vaccinations.

◆ Repeat any unexpected viral load result.

◆ Two measurements 1 month apart should be done before making any significant clinical care change if the change is based on the viral load.

◆ Ideally, repeat tests should be done in the same laboratory using the same method of testing.

Height, weight and clinical wellbeing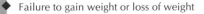

Special attention needs to be directed towards monitoring the growth, and physical and neurological development of the child. The child should also be examined for signs of ARV drug toxicity *(see table on page 185)*.

The following indications are suggestive of progressive HIV disease:

◆ Failure to gain weight or loss of weight

◆ A delay in milestones

◆ Infections such as TB

A 'road to health' or growth monitoring chart is a valuable tool for measuring growth in children under 5 years of age.

◆ ART and care

Monitoring programme – clinic visits and consultations

At the beginning of ART the following tests should be done:

◆ CD4 cell count

◆ HIV viral load

The following issues need to be thoroughly discussed with the primary caregiver:

◆ The clinical outlook for the child (prognosis)

◆ The treatment plan

◆ The need for strict adherence to therapy

◆ How and when to administer the drugs

◆ The need for regular follow-up visits

◆ The cost

◆ The need for drugs to be given for life

◆ Show actual drugs to the caregiver and explain carefully how and when they should be given

1 – 2 weeks after starting ART

◆ Make a follow-up appointment to discuss how the child is tolerating the medication and drug adherence.

4 weeks after starting ART

◆ Examine the child for signs of drug toxicity, and do blood tests for signs of toxicity (FBC, liver function).

3 months after starting ART

◆ Do a general examination of the child looking for signs of drug toxicity.

◆ Do blood tests for signs of toxicity (FBC, liver function).

◆ Repeat the CD4 and viral load blood tests.

◆ Reinforce issues of adherence, and potential drug side effects and toxicity to the caregiver.

Thereafter, 4 – 6 monthly clinical reviews

◆ Continue to see the child every 3 months until viral load and CD4 cell counts are stable and drug tolerance has been established. The child can then be reviewed every 4 – 6 months.

◆ ART in babies under the age of 3 months

ART should be considered when there is an early diagnosis of HIV infection. This is when HIV infection is confirmed in a baby less than 3 months of age by a positive HIV PCR test and a viral load assessment.

Babies under the age of 3 months are often in the 'primary HIV infection' phase. It is possible to achieve viral suppression and normal immunity.

The following are important considerations:

◆ Viral levels are usually very high and 4 drugs are often needed

◆ Long-term toxicity of the drugs

◆ Viral resistance to the drugs

◆ Cost of the drugs on an ongoing long-term basis

A decision to start therapy in babies under 3 months of age should not be taken lightly. It should be undertaken in consultation with colleagues and caregivers.

Babies under 3 months of age often have very high viral loads. Aggressive ART is needed to achieve adequate viral outcomes (low viral loads) and immunological outcomes (stable or elevated CD4 cell counts).

CHILDREN WITH HIV/AIDS

The current drugs used in babies under the age of 3 months:

CATEGORY I (NRTI – thymidine base)	CATEGORY II (NRTI – other)	CATEGORY III (NNRTI)	CATEGORY IV (PI)	CATEGORY V (NRTI – new)
◆ Stavudine (d4T) ◆ Zidovudine (ZDV)	◆ Didanosine (ddI) ◆ Lamivudine (3TC)	◆ Nevirapine (NVP)	◆ Ritonavir (RTV) ◆ Nelfinavir (NFV)	◆ Abacavir (ABC)

Recommended ARV drug options in babies

◆ 3 NRTIs (1 from Category I; 1 from Category II; and ABC from Category V)
  PLUS 1 PI (from Category IV)

◆ 3 NRTIs (1 from Category I; 1 from Category II; and ABC from Category V)
  PLUS NVP (from Category III)

◆ 2 NRTIs (1 from Category I; 1 from Category II)
  PLUS 1 PI (from Category IV)
  PLUS NVP (from Category III)

Note: If 4 drugs are not possible (cost, toxicity etc.) a 3-drug regimen could be considered *(see page 181 under recommended ARV drug options in children)*.

The drug dosages for babies under 3 months of age

Drug	Formulation	Dosage
NRTIs		
Zidovudine (ZDV) Retrovir®	Susp. 10 mg / ml	4 mg / kg 3 x daily until 29 days, then 160 mg / m^2 3 x daily
Didanosine (ddI) Videx®	Susp. 10 mg / ml Tabs 25 mg	50 mg / m^2 2 x daily
Stavudine (D4T) Zerit®	Susp. 1 mg / ml	< 29 days: 0,5 mg / kg 2 x daily > 30 days: 1 mg / kg 2 x daily
Abacavir (ABC) Ziagen®	Susp. 20 mg / ml	8 mg / kg 2 x daily
Lamivudine (3TC®)	Susp. 10 mg / ml	< 1 month: 2 mg / kg 2 x daily > 1 month: 4 mg / kg 2 x daily
NNRTIs		
Nevirapine Viramune®	Susp. 10 mg / ml	5 mg / kg / day x 14 days; then 120 mg / m^2 2 x daily x 14 days; then 200 mg / m^2 2 x daily
PIs		
Ritonavir (RTV) Norvir®	Susp. 80 mg / ml	> 1 month 450 mg / m^2 2 x daily
Nelfinavir (NFV) Vira-cept®	Powder 50 mg / g Tabs 250 mg	55 – 65 mg / kg 2 x daily

Source: 'Antiretroviral therapy in children.' Southern African Journal of HIV Medicine, October 2002, page 29

CHILDREN WITH HIV/AIDS

◆ ART for children over the age of 3 months

ART should be considered when a child is diagnosed at a later stage because of:

– development of HIV-related symptomatic disease

– or because of a positive HIV diagnosis in the mother

The current drugs used in children over the age of 3 months:

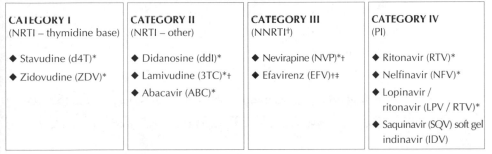

CATEGORY I (NRTI – thymidine base)	CATEGORY II (NRTI – other)	CATEGORY III (NNRTI†)	CATEGORY IV (PI)
◆ Stavudine (d4T)* ◆ Zidovudine (ZDV)*	◆ Didanosine (ddI)* ◆ Lamivudine (3TC)*† ◆ Abacavir (ABC)*	◆ Nevirapine (NVP)*† ◆ Efavirenz (EFV)†‡	◆ Ritonavir (RTV)* ◆ Nelfinavir (NFV)* ◆ Lopinavir / ritonavir (LPV / RTV)* ◆ Saquinavir (SQV) soft gel indinavir (IDV)

* Available in paediatric formulations.
† Require single mutation for development of resistance. Some experts therefore only use them in regimens with a good chance of attaining undetectable viral loads.
‡ Efavirenz (EFV) is only available in capsule form. There are no data for children under 3 years of age.

Source: 'Antiretroviral therapy in children.' Southern African Journal of HIV Medicine, October 2002, page 29

Recommended ARV drug options in children

Preferred regimens

◆ 2 NRTIs (1 from Category I; 1 from Category II) **or** (3TC + ABC from Category II)
PLUS 1 PI (from Category IV)
e.g. ZDV + 3TC + RTV **or** 3TC + ABC + RTV

◆ 2 NRTIs (1 drug from Category I; 1 from Category II) **or** (3TC + ABC from Category II)
PLUS 1 NNRTI (from Category III)
e.g. d4T (or ZDV) + ddI (or 3TC) **or** ABC + 3TC + NVP **or** EFV

EFV and NVP develop resistance rapidly if viral suppression is not excellent (undetectable viral loads). These drugs should only be used for viral loads < 150 000 copies / mm³.

Alternative regimens

◆ 1 NRTI (from Category I or II)
PLUS 1 NNRTI (from Category III)
PLUS 1 PI (from Category IV)

◆ For children with low viral loads:
ABC **plus** ZDV **plus** 3TC

Dual therapies

In situations where resources are limited the following dual therapies are recommended. However, it must be noted that these are sub-optimal with a higher likelihood of drug resistance. They may be considered in children with less severe disease. They should probably not be used in children with very high viral levels.

- ◆ d4T **plus** ddI
- ◆ ZDV **plus** ddI
- ◆ ZDV **plus** 3TC
- ◆ d4T **plus** 3TC

The drug dosages for children

Drug	Formulations	Dosage (per dose)	Frequency	Storage	Comments
NRTIs					
Zidovudine (ZDV) Retrovir®	Susp. 10 mg / ml Caps 100 mg, 250 mg Tabs 300 mg	90 – 180 mg / m² 180 mg / m²	8 hourly 12 hourly	Room temperature	
Didanosine (ddI) Videx®	Susp. 10 mg / ml Tabs 25 mg, 50 mg, 100 mg, 150 mg	90 – 120 mg / m²	12 hourly Can give total daily dose x 1 in older children	Refrigerate suspension	Half an hour before meals or 1 hour after meals. Use single daily dose if necessary for adherence.
Stavudine (d4T) Zerit®	Susp. 1 mg / ml Caps 20 mg, 30 mg, 40 mg	1 mg / kg	12 hourly	Refrigerate suspension	Capsules stable in water suspension for 24 hours in refrigerator.
Abacavir Ziagen®	Susp. 20 mg / ml Tabs 300 mg	8 mg / kg	12 hourly	Room temperature	**Watch for hypersensitivity reaction. Do not rechallenge after hypersensitivity reaction.**
Lamivudine (3TC®)	Susp. 10 mg / ml Tabs 150 mg	4 mg / kg	12 hourly	Room temperature	
NNRTIs					
Nevirapine Viramune®	Susp. 10 mg / ml Tabs 200 mg	120 – 200 mg / m² Start at 120 mg / m² daily for 14 days and increase to 2 x daily if no rash or severe side-effects.	12 hourly	Room temperature	Skin rash usually occurs in 1st 6 weeks. Do not increase dosage until rash disappears. **Watch for liver toxicity.**
Efavirenz Stocrin®	Caps 50 and 200 mg (susp. available from manufacturer)	13 – < 15 kg: 200 mg 15 – < 20 kg: 250 mg 20 – < 25 kg: 300 mg 25 – < 32,5 kg: 350 mg 32,5 – < 40 kg: 400 mg > 40 kg: 600 mg	daily	Room temperature	No data < 3 yrs and < 13 kg. Give at night to avoid CNS side-effects.

PIs					
Ritonavir Norvir®	Susp. 80 mg / ml	Start at 250 mg / m² / dose. Increase by 50 mg / m² every 2 – 3 days up to 400 mg / m². If < 2 yrs of age give 450 mg / m²	12 hourly		Take with food. Bitter; coat mouth with peanut butter or give with chocolate milk. Take 2 hours apart from ddl.
Nelfinavir Vira-cept®	Susp. 50 mg / 1 g spoon and 200 mg per teaspoon Tabs 250 mg	Paediatric: 55 mg / kg (adolescent: 750 mg 3 x daily or 1 250 mg 2 x daily). Some experts use 35 – 45 mg / kg 3 x daily > 2 yrs of age and 45 – 55 mg / kg 3 x daily < 2 yrs of age	12 hourly		Give 2 hours before or 1 hour after ddl. Best with light meal. Do not use with rifampicin. Powder is 5% active drug and the rest is carrier powder. Most experts prefer to crush the tablets and suspend in milk or water, or sprinkle on pudding.
Lopinavir / ritonavir Kaletra®	Oral solution 80 mg lopinavir (LPV) and 20 mg ritonavir (RTV) per ml Caps 133 mg LPV / 33 mg RTV	Patients not taking NVP or EFV give 230 mg LPV component / m² (max. 400 mg LPV = adolescent dose). Patients taking NVP or EFV or ART experienced give 300 mg LPV component / m² (max. 533 mg LPV = adolescent dose).	12 hourly	Oral solution and capsules should be refrigerated. Can be kept at room temperature up to 25°C if used within 2 months.	Administer with food. High-fat meal increases absorption, especially of the liquid preparation. If co-administered with ddl, ddl should be given 1 hour before or 2 hours after lopinavir / ritonavir.
Saquinavir Invirase® – hard gel capsule	Hard gel caps (HGC) 200 mg (only use together with RTV)	Single PI (SGC only) – 50 mg / kg. Dual PIs - give SQV 50 mg / mg RTV 100 mg / m²	8 hourly 12 hourly 12 hourly		Administer within 2 hours after a full meal to increase absorption. Sun exposure can cause photosensitivity reactions; therefore, sunscreen or protective clothing is recommended.
Fortovase® – soft gel capsule	Soft gel caps (SGC) 200 mg	Adolescent 1 200 mg or 1 600 mg	8 hourly 12 hourly		

Body surface area (m2) = $\sqrt{\text{height (cm) x weight (kg)}} \div 60$

Source: 'Antiretroviral therapy in children.' Southern African Journal of HIV Medicine, October 2002, page 30

◆ **Important points about ART**

◆ The following drug interactions are known:
  – Efavirenz causes reduced levels of clarithromycin.
  – Do not use ritonavir with cisapride, midazolam and some other drugs (check package insert).
  – Rifampicin leads to reduced levels of indinavir, nelfinavir and saquinavir.

◆ 3TC resistance develops more easily than other NRTI drugs. Therefore 3TC should only be used in combinations of 3 drugs.

CHILDREN WITH HIV/AIDS

◆ NRTIs may cause lactic acidosis – a rare but life-threatening condition resulting from mitochondrial damage *(see also page 90).*

◆ Rifampicin may interact with PIs and the NNRTIs. The following options can be considered:
  – Delay the start of ART until TB treatment is complete.
  – With severe HIV disease, delay ART for 1 month after starting TB treatment *(see also page 255).*
  – Use a regimen that is compatible with rifampicin, e.g. 2 NRTIs **plus** ritonavir or EFV (if older than 3 months).
  – Use 3 NRTIs, e.g. ZDV / 3TC / ABC (in situations of low viral loads).
  – Use rifabutin (expensive option) instead of rifampicin. Avoid using ritonavir if using rifabutin.
  – In children with TB who start ART, there can be an unusual or paradoxical worsening of the TB disease due to an immune reconstitution disease. For this reason it is often best to start TB treatment at least 2 months before starting ART. In children with less severe immune-deficiency, it is best to delay ART until completion of the TB treatment *(see also pages 90 and 255).*

◆ ART outcomes

Successful ART should achieve the following:

◆ A significant reduction in viral load. Ideally this should reduce to less than 400 copies / mm^3. A decline of at least 1 log (10-fold reduction) is usually considered successful.

◆ The CD4 cell count and percentage should ideally improve, or at least remain stable if it was previously declining steadily.

◆ Opportunistic infections such as thrush, diarrhoea, recurrent respiratory infections, and skin infections should decline in severity and frequency. They should ideally disappear and remain absent.

◆ Health status should improve – wellness, weight gain, fitness.

ART has failed if the following are present:

◆ Severe opportunistic infections continue and do not reduce in severity or frequency.

◆ The CD4 cell count continues to drop.

◆ Viral load does not drop to significantly lower levels or is not maintained at these low levels.

◆ Other indicators of illness or poor health status continue such as weight loss, failure to thrive etc.

If treatment failure occurs, there is drug resistance, or poor adherence or tolerance to the drugs. Treatment failure needs to be investigated, and the appropriate course of action taken. If there is drug resistance or drug intolerance, change the regimen. If there is poor adherence, then steps must be taken to improve and monitor adherence.

◆ Possible side effects of ARV drugs

Class	Drug	Side effects / toxicity
NRTIs		
	ZDV (Retrovir®)	Anaemia, granulocytopenia, myopathy, lactic acidosis
	ddl (Videx®)	Common: abdominal pain, nausea, vomiting Uncommon: pancreatitis, peripheral neuropathy, lactic acidosis
	Stavudine (Zerit®)	Common: headache, rash, gastro-intestinal symptoms Uncommon: pancreatitis, peripheral neuropathy, lactic acidosis
	Abacavir (Ziagen®)	Hypersensitivity reaction (with or without rash – may be fatal in adults and children), fever, rash, fatigue, nausea, vomiting, diarrhoea, pharyngitis, dyspnoea, cough, elevated ALT, creatinine or CPK, lymphopenia lactic acidosis
	Lamivudine (3TC®)	Common: headache, fatigue, abdominal pain Uncommon: pancreatitis, peripheral neuropathy, lactic acidosis
NNRTIs		
	Nevirapine (Viramune®)	**Skin rash**, sedative effect, diarrhoea, **liver toxicity**
	Efavirenz (Stocrin®)	Skin rash, CNS problems (sleep disturbance, confusion, abnormal thinking), teratogenic in primates
PIs		
	Ritonavir (Norvir®)	Nausea, vomiting, diarrhoea, hypercholesterolaemia, hypertriglyceridaemia
	Nelfinavir (Vira-cept®)	Diarrhoea, exacerbated chronic liver disease, hypercholesterolaemia, hypertriglyceridaemia
Ribo-nucleotide reductase inhibitors		
	Hydroxyurea (Hydrea®)	Granulocytopenia, anaemia Withdrawn from ARV studies because of reports of fatal pancreatitis in patients on combination therapy; Side effects more common in patients with advanced disease

Source: 'Antiretroviral therapy in children.' Southern African Journal of HIV Medicine, October 2002, page 32

◆ Changing ARV drugs

◆ If this is necessary due to drug side-effects or toxicity, a simple substitution from the categories listed above can be made.

◆ If drug resistance is present, at least 2 drugs should be changed.

It is best to consult an HIV-experienced paediatrician in the above situations.

Recognising and treating
HIV-associated infections and conditions

It is very important to recognise and treat any infection as early as possible. The parents and childcarers must be encouraged **to seek medical help as soon as possible** if the child develops any unusual signs or symptoms.

Hospital admissions are an additional risk for HIV-infected children who are immune-deficient. The hospital environment exposes children to many harmful pathogens (germs) which can be dangerous to children with low immunity. Before admitting a child to hospital, you must consider this high-risk environment.

Indications for admission include:

◆ An acutely ill child who is seriously ill or whose life is at risk

◆ The need for specific observations

◆ Oxygen therapy; parenteral therapy; IV fluid therapy

◆ Naso-gastric feeding

In *Chapter 7* the management of the most common HIV-related conditions in adults is discussed. Where appropriate children should be treated in a similar way. *Some of the more common conditions are outlined below:*

Orral thrush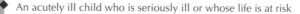

Treatment

℞

You can use any of the following in order of strength and cost:

◆ Gentian violet 1% applied locally

◆ Nystatin/clotrimazole 1%, oral suspension 1 – 2 mls applied locally, 4 – 6 times a day

◆ Ketoconazole 3 – 6 mg/kg daily orally for 7 days

◆ Fluconazole 3 mg/kg daily orally for 7 days

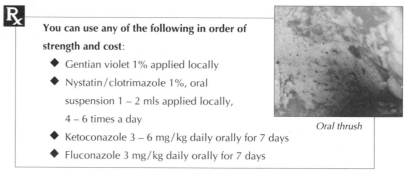
Oral thrush

Diarrhoea

Diarrhoea may be due to:

◆ Protozoal infections, such as giardia, entamoeba

◆ Bacterial infections, such as salmonella, shigella, campylobacter

◆ Viral infections, such as rotavirus, cytomegalovirus

◆ Fungi – candidiasis

◆ Worm infestation

Treatment

℞

Treat the diarrhoea as follows:

◆ **Oral hydration fluids** should be given for diarrhoeal disease. Also make sure that the mother knows how to make a home-made oral hydration solution. She should know what fluid to give and how to use it.

◆ You should advise her to use **any fluid that is available**, such as rice-water, porridge-water, soups, teas etc. Home-made oral hydration fluids are ideal *(see next page)*.

◆ **Watch out for signs of dehydration**.
These may include:
  – dry mouth, eyes and skin
  – poor skin elasticity
  – poor urine output
  – sunken fontanelle and eyes
  – rapid pulse and breathing
  – shock and coma in severe dehydration

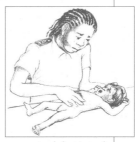

Look for signs of dehydration

Refer children with severe dehydration to hospital for intravenous fluids.

◆ **Give nutritional and electrolyte supplements** in severe or ongoing diarrhoea.

◆ **Drug treatment**
  – antibiotics, such as Nalidixic acid (50 mg / kg / day), can be tried if the diarrhoea is bloody.
  – other antibiotics which may be beneficial include co-trimoxazole ampicillin, chloramphenicol and erythromycin. (Antibiotics must be used with care.)
  – metronidazole (Flagyl) 30 mg / kg / day for 5 days is recommended for giardia or amoebic causes of diarrhoea.
  – thiabendazole 50 mg / kg 12 hourly for 2 days for worm infestation.

Note: Hospitalisation should be avoided unless oral rehydration fails. The use of anti-diarrhoeal medications should be avoided, as it has been proved that they do not work. Ongoing dehydrating diarrhoea is an indication for changing milk feeds, but only if such formulae are readily available. It is essential that children receive adequate nutrition during and after the episode of diarrhoea.

A good home-made oral hydration fluid

- ◆ 1 cup of water
- ◆ 2 teaspoons of sugar
- ◆ 2 finger pinches of salt
- ◆ Some fresh orange or other juice for taste and potassium replacement

or

- ◆ 1 litre of water
- ◆ 5 teaspoons of sugar
- ◆ ½ teaspoon of salt
- ◆ Fresh fruit juice for taste

The child should be given at least one cup of this fluid after every stool.

Tuberculosis

TB is a common HIV-related disease. It may be pulmonary, extra-pulmonary or miliary. Children with miliary, severe pulmonary disease or tuberculous meningitis should be treated in hospital. Children with other forms of tuberculosis must be placed on an initial two month **intensive phase** of treatment.

The **continuation phase** for children with primary TB, and / or effusion, is 2 months. For children with progressive primary, cavitating or non-pulmonary TB, the continuation phase is 4 months *(see table below)*. In all cases attempt to obtain specimens for smear, culture and sensitivity.

Treatment of children with TB (other than tuberculous meningitis or miliary TB)

Intensive Phase (2 months)	5 – 10 kg	11 – 20 kg	21 – 30 kg
Rifampicin / INH Combination tablet (150 / 100 mg)	½ tab	1 tab	2 tabs
Pyrazinamide 500 mg	½ tab	1 tab	2 tabs
Continuation Phase (2 – 4 months)	**5 – 10 kg**	**11 – 20 kg**	**21 – 30 kg**
Rifampicin / INH Combination tablet (150 / 100 mg)	½ tab	1 tab	2 tabs

Source: S.A Tuberculosis Control Programme: Practical Guidelines 1996

See page 184 for special considerations when using ARV in children with TB.

Bacterial and respiratory infections

Signs of respiratory distress

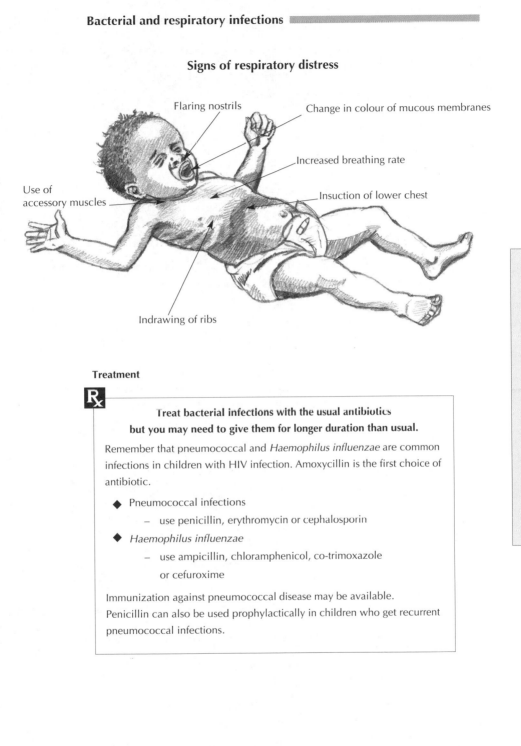

Flaring nostrils

Change in colour of mucous membranes

Increased breathing rate

Use of accessory muscles

Insuction of lower chest

Indrawing of ribs

Treatment

Rx

> **Treat bacterial infections with the usual antibiotics**
> **but you may need to give them for longer duration than usual.**
>
> Remember that pneumococcal and *Haemophilus influenzae* are common infections in children with HIV infection. Amoxycillin is the first choice of antibiotic.
>
> ◆ Pneumococcal infections
>   – use penicillin, erythromycin or cephalosporin
> ◆ *Haemophilus influenzae*
>   – use ampicillin, chloramphenicol, co-trimoxazole or cefuroxime
>
> Immunization against pneumococcal disease may be available. Penicillin can also be used prophylactically in children who get recurrent pneumococcal infections.

Pneumocystis carinii pneumonia (PCP)

PCP is one of the common severe opportunistic infections found in children with HIV infection.

PCP may be suspected if there is:

◆ Sudden onset fever

◆ Tachypnoea and cyanosis

◆ A diffuse interstitial infiltrate on X-ray

If PCP is suspected, refer to hospital.

Treatment

℞

◆ Co-trimoxazole (20 mg / kg / day of the trimethoprim component) in 4 divided doses for 14 – 21 days.

◆ Steroids (2 mg / kg / day) are also recommended.

◆ Since bacterial infection is often a co-infection, broad-spectrum antibiotics are also recommended e.g. ampicillin and gentamicin or a cephalosporin).

Lymphoid interstitial pneumonitis (LIP)

This is an unusual respiratory disease found in HIV-infected children. The child usually develops an ongoing cough with mild wheezing. Chest X-ray usually shows reticular or nodular interstitial infiltrates and mediastinal lymphadenipathy.

Treatment

℞

◆ Treat with steroids – 2 mg / kg / day for 10 – 14 days.

◆ However the benefit of steroids is not certain.

Failure to thrive

Common causes include diarrhoea, tuberculosis, recurrent infections and HIV infection itself.

Treatment

℞

This depends on any identifiable cause

◆ Provide adequate nutritional and vitamin supplements.

◆ Treat any underlying conditions.

Skin conditions

The treatment of common skin conditions is discussed on page 137. (Paediatric doses need to be given for children.)

Oral candidiasis

Oral candidiasis is very common in HIV-infected children.

Treatment

- ◆ Nystatin suspension (1 ml 4 x daily)

- ◆ Or daktarin gel (apply every 4 – 6 hours)

If no response, or if severe infection treat with:

- ◆ Oral ketaconazole 3 – 6 mg / kg / day for 7 days

- ◆ Or fluconazole 3 mg / kg / day orally until clear

Anaemia and other blood disorders

Treatment

- ◆ Elemental iron 2 – 6 mg / kg given daily in three divided doses.

- ◆ Folate 2,5 mg should be given weekly.

Children with easy bruising or bleeding should be referred for assessment.

Neurological conditions

Neurological conditions include acute episodes of infection, such as meningitis or encephalitis and encephelopathies.

Treatment

- ◆ Meningitis is diagnosed and treated as usual. Remember to think of more chronic forms of meningitis, such as tuberculosis or Cryptococcal meningitis.

- ◆ Refer children with signs of neurological disorders to the local paediatric centre for assessment and care.

Preventing opportunistic infections

Preventing opportunistic infections is an important feature in caring for children with HIV i.e. children with low CD4 counts or with advanced HIV disease, as shown by repeated infections, recurrent oral thrush, failure to thrive etc.

◆ Prophylaxis against some important and severe opportunistic infections

It is important to know when to begin prophylactic therapy.

This is determined by:

◆ The immune status of the child

◆ The prevalence and severity of the inter-current infection

◆ The efficacy of the intervention

◆ The cost of the intervention

Prophylaxis can be considered for:

◆ Candida

◆ *Pneumocystis carinii* pneumonia

◆ TB

◆ Recurrent bacterial infections

◆ Toxoplasmosis

Candida (thrush) prophylaxis

◆ Give anti-candida (thrush) medication on a daily basis
e.g. gentian violet, mycostatin (Nystatin) 100,000 IU 6 – 12 hourly.

◆ *See page 134 for more details. (Give paediatric doses where appropriate.)*

Pneumocystis carinii pneumonia (PCP) prophylaxis

The risk of PCP is greatest in the first year of life.

℞

- Babies born to HIV-positive women, should start co-trimoxazole prophylaxis at 4 weeks, and continue until 1 year of age.

- Where PCR HIV testing is available this should be performed at 3 – 4 months of age. If PCR negative, prophylaxis should be stopped. If PCR positive, prophylaxis should be continued until the child is 1 year old.

After 1 year of age prophylaxis should be given when the CD4 cell count falls below the age adjusted norm (*see table on page 174*). If CD4 levels are not available, all symptomatic children should receive prophylaxis (Clinical Categories B and C – *see pages 169 – 171*) .

The recommended drug is co-trimoxazole given 3 times a week (Monday, Tuesday and Wednesday) in the following doses:

Weight	Dose of co-trimoxazole
< 5 kg	5 ml
5 – 9,9 kg	7,5 ml
10 – 14,9 kg	10 ml
15 – 21,9 kg	15 ml or 1,5 tabs
> 22 kg	20 ml or 2 tabs

Tuberculosis prophylaxis

There is a close association between HIV infection and TB.

℞

Prophylaxis should be given to all children with a positive TB contact once active disease has been excluded.

The recommended regimen is described below.

Children under 2 years of age

Give prophylaxis for 3 months only.

Weight	Dose rifampicin / INH (150 / 100 mg) tablet
< 5 kg	¼ tablet
5 – 10 kg	½ tablet
11 – 20 kg	1 tablet

Children over 2 years of age

Give prophylaxis for 6 months with INH only.

Weight	Dose INH
10 – 20 kg	100 mg
21 – 30 kg	200 mg

Source: The SA Tuberculosis Control Programme Practical Guidelines (1996)

Recurrent bacterial infection prophylaxis

Recurrent bacterial infections are common problems in HIV-positive children, and not always related to immune-deficiency.

If recurrent bacterial infection is a problem consider the following:

℞

◆ Immunoglobulin (400 mg / kg monthly) can be used to prevent infections. It is however:
  – not widely available;
  – very expensive;
  – of limited benefit in children who are already on co-trimoxazole.

◆ H influenza B and pneumococcal vaccines are of benefit for these organisms (*see also pages 199 – 200*).

◆ Co-trimoxazole is an effective prophylactic for a variety of bacterial and protozoan infections. As it is also indicated for the prevention of PCP, it is recommended that the same drug dose (*see previous page*) be used for the prevention of recurrent bacterial infections.

Measles and chickenpox prophylaxis

If an immune-deficient child is exposed to measles or chickenpox, consider giving the following:

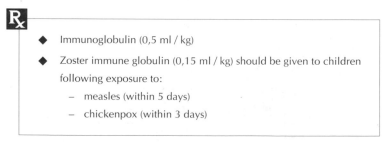

℞

◆ Immunoglobulin (0,5 ml / kg)

◆ Zoster immune globulin (0,15 ml / kg) should be given to children following exposure to:
  – measles (within 5 days)
  – chickenpox (within 3 days)

◆ Nutritional education and support

Malnutrition adversely affects immunity. It also makes children more prone to opportunistic infections.

Deficiencies of many micronutrients, including those which are essential for normal immune-function, make the HIV condition worse. Vitamin A deficiency is common and makes children more prone to infections.

Supplementation with Vitamin A has:

◆ Significant short-term improvements in immune function

◆ Reduced morbidity, particularly in relation to diarrhoeal disease

The management of children at risk for malnutrition should therefore include:

◆ Growth monitoring

◆ Dietary advice

◆ Ensuring adequate nutrient intake

◆ Ensuring adequate intake of micro-nutrients – Vitamin A, iron and folate. Vitamin A supplementation is recommended on a six monthly basis as follows:

    – under 6 months of age – 50 000 IU

    – 6 – 12 months of age – 100 000 IU

    – 1 year and older – 200 000 IU

Where suitable Vitamin A preparations are not available, a daily multivitamin preparation containing Vitamin A (usually about 5 000 IU) should be prescribed. Children who are anaemic should receive iron and folate.

◆ Treatment of nutritional-related infections

    – candidiasis and parasites such as ascaris (round worms) and trichuris (whipworms) must be treated

    – from the age of 1 year all children should receive a course of albendazole every 6 months for the treatment of intestinal worms.

◆ The method of infant feeding – breast or formula (*see Chapter 10*)

Hospitalisation of children with HIV/AIDS

Most HIV-related conditions and general care can and should be done at the primary care level. Hospital admissions must be carefully considered. HIV-infected children admitted to hospital should not be unnecessarily isolated.

However immune-deficient children may need to be kept away from other in-patients who have infectious conditions.

◆ Guide as to when to refer children with HIV/AIDS for hospital care:

- ◆ An acutely, severely ill child e.g. respiratory, gastro-enteritis, TB, neurological problems etc.

- ◆ A child not responding to treatment of any serious clinical problem

- ◆ A suspected PCP or LIP

- ◆ An unexplained, persistent pyrexia (for investigation if tests are not available at primary level)

- ◆ Unusual complications where treatment is not available at primary level

- ◆ For investigations not available at primary level

- ◆ Continued and severe weight loss

- ◆ For special nursing or treatment needs (e.g. blood transfusion, drip, intravenous therapy)

- ◆ For an initial assessment of certain conditions such as chronic lung disease, persistent diarrhoea and recurrent sepsis. These children can then be followed up at primary level care.

> **Hospitals are risky places for children with poor immune systems. Referral and admission to hospital must be carefully considered.**

◆ Terminal and palliative child care

Children who are in a very terminal phase of the disease may benefit more from palliative care rather than very costly intensive care. This may serve only to prolong the pain and discomfort without adding to the quality of life.

There are decisions which need to be jointly made with parents, and other caregivers. Each child's situation must be considered with regard to withdrawing or withholding definitive / curative treatment.

The decision to provide palliative care should be based on the following:

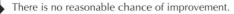

- ◆ There is no reasonable chance of improvement.

- ◆ There is no purpose to the management.

- ◆ The status is unbearable for the child / family.

- ◆ The child has an acute HIV encephalopathy and / or severe HIV-related wasting syndrome.

Once such a decision has been taken, every effort should be made to provide palliative care. The child must be kept comfortable and must feel that he / she is loved and cared for. This includes oxygen, morphine, naso-gastric feeds and maximum support aimed at comfort but excludes antibiotics. Many parents prefer that their children die at home, and their wishes should be respected. Terminal care should ideally be provided on a home-care basis with support from primary care and other facilities.

Children do not readily talk about their fears and worries. They need to be carefully counselled and reassured.

Care for terminally ill patients is discussed in more detail in Chapter 14.

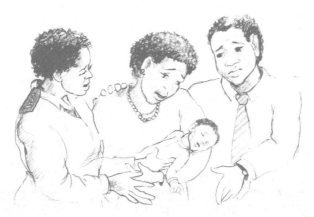

Counselling and support

Most children with HIV / AIDS will be under the age of 5 years.

Occasionally an older child may have become infected from a blood transfusion or from being sexually abused.

Children, or their siblings, may suffer from stigmatisation and discrimination. Strict confidentiality of a child's HIV infection is very important.

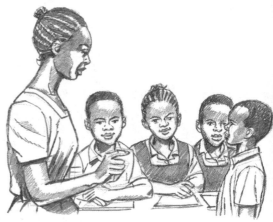

You may need to reassure the local school or day care officials if there is any discrimination or rejection towards a child or his/her siblings.

Counselling and support for the parents or care-giver are an essential part of your therapy.

Often the parents are also HIV-positive and you may need to care for them as well. Parenting an HIV-positive child may be very stressful and depressing. Older brothers and sisters may also need counselling during the illness or after the death of the sibling. You may also need to get assistance from social workers, child welfare officers, or refer the family to other agencies for support and advice.

Children with HIV / AIDS must be encouraged and allowed to live as normal a social life as possible. They must not be excluded from usual activities.

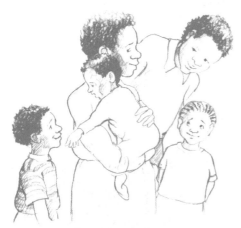

Children, in normal circumstances, do not pass on the virus to other children and parents should be reassured that their child is not infectious to other children.

HIV-infected children should be accepted into schools, crèches, nursery schools, day-care centres etc. unless they are ill and unable to attend for medical reasons. Immuno-suppressed children may also come into contact with many childhood infections at the child-care centres, crèches, schools, clinics, etc. This may need to be considered if the child is getting repeated infections.

Avoid hospital admissions unless the admission is essential. Try to keep children with HIV infection at home and with their families as much as possible.

Immunisation of children with HIV infection

All the usual childhood vaccines can be given to children with HIV infection as per the schedule below

Children with HIV infection should be fully immunised. Many children with AIDS die of diseases which can be prevented by immunisation.

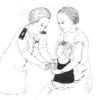

Immunisation

Give the full course of vaccines to the HIV-infected or HIV-positive child if the child is well and does not have any signs and symptoms of advanced HIV infection.

Children born to HIV-infected mothers can be given BCG at birth. If there are signs of advanced HIV disease in the child, then you should **not** give the BCG vaccine.

There have been reports of BCG disease in HIV-positive children. Recommendations for BCG in HIV-positive babies may change.

HiB vaccine has been incorporated into the national immunisation programme.

If available, pneumococcal and influenzae vaccines should also be considered (*see below*). However the effectiveness of these in HIV-infected children is not yet certain.

> **Children with HIV infection must be fully immunised.**

Standard Immunisation Schedule

Age	Vaccine*
Birth	BCG, OPV
6 weeks	DTP, HBV, HiB, OPV
10 weeks	DTP, HBV, HiB, OPV
14 weeks	DTP, HBV, HiB, OPV
9 months	Measles (MMR if available)
18 months	Measles, DTP
4 – 5 years	OPV, DT

*BCG = Bacille Calmette-Guérin (TB)
OPV = Oral polio
DTP = Diphtheria, Tetanus, Pertussis
HiB = Haemophilus Influenza type B
HBV = Hepatitis B
MMR = Mumps, Measles, Rubella

◆ Information on some of the recommended immunisations

DTP and HiB

 ◆ It is now possible to get a DTP and HiB vaccine combined.

Influenzae

◆ The annually updated influenzae vaccine is recommended.

◆ It should be administered in time to provide adequate protection before the commencement of cold weather.

Pneumococcal vaccine

◆ A single dose of polyvalent Pneumococcal vaccine should be administered to children with HIV infection.

◆ It is only recommended for children over two years of age.

Hepatitis B vaccine (HBV)

◆ This can also be considered if not already given.

BCG vaccine

◆ Remember that TB is common in adults and children with HIV infection. The brothers and sisters of HIV-positive children, or children of HIV-positive parents, should all be immunised with BCG.

◆ Give BCG to the children or their siblings if they have not been previously immunised or if their PPD skin test is negative.

◆ Recent reports of BCG disease in babies with HIV infection may lead to changes in BCG immunisation recommendations.

Avoid immunising the child with live vaccines if the child is very ill. Rather delay the immunisation until the child has improved.

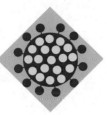

Chapter 9

WOMEN WITH HIV INFECTION AND AIDS

The spread of HIV infection in women

The clinical course of HIV/AIDS in women

The effect of HIV on women's health

The effect of HIV on pregnancy and childbirth

Contraception for women with HIV infection

Prophylaxis after sexual exposure

The spread of HIV infection in women

In Africa, HIV infection has been spreading more rapidly in women than in men.

Some of the reasons why women are at higher risk for acquiring HIV infection and how this affects them and their health will be discussed in this chapter.

Pregnancy and HIV infection is another very important aspect to consider, as women often find out that they have HIV infection during pregnancy. Approximately 30% of HIV-infected women pass on the infection to their children. This may take place during pregnancy, childbirth or while breast feeding. Mother to child transmission and its prevention is also discussed in *Chapter 10.*

◆ Why are women vulnerable to HIV infection?

Women are often more vulnerable to HIV infection than men. There are many socio-economic reasons why they are more exposed to the HIV virus. Also any condition causing inflammation or damage to the lining of the genital tract helps the HIV virus gain entry into the body.

Some of the more common reasons why women are so vulnerable include:

Receptive sexual partner

◆ A woman is the receptive partner during sex. Infected semen is deposited in the woman's vagina and remains there for some time, which gives the virus an opportunity to gain entry into the body.

Uterine, cervical and vaginal conditions which promote HIV transmission

◆ Many women have **cervical conditions**, such as erosions, cervical ectopy, sexually transmitted diseases (STIs) and occasionally cervical cancers.

◆ **Inflammation** or damage to the vaginal walls. This is usually from STIs or from the use of herbal and other substances used in the vagina. Spermicidal preparations may also cause inflammation. The HIV virus has an attraction to many of the inflammatory types of cells.

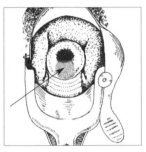

Cervican erosion

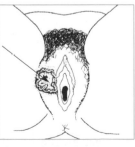

Chancroid ulcer

◆ **STIs often go unnoticed** or hidden in women and they may not seek treatment. Also in low socio-economic areas there is often poor access to health care to get treatment for STIs and other genital diseases.

◆ **Menstruation** also results in a large, raw, exposed area of the inner uterine lining which may make the transmission of HIV easier just before, during or after menstruating.

Status of women

The following factors help to expose women and girls to HIV and other STIs more frequently.

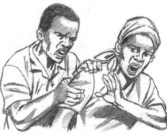

◆ The social status of women, especially in low socio-economic communities, often results in women having less control over their sexual lives.

They also have less control negotiating safer sexual practices with their sexual partners. They are often forced into unwanted sexual encounters because of life circumstances e.g. they may have to resort to selling sex for much-needed money for basic life necessities, such as food and shelter. Women may also need to leave home and seek work elsewhere, thereby leaving their husbands, boyfriends and usual sexual partners.

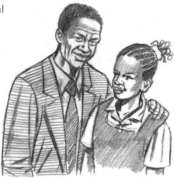

◆ Women are also more vulnerable to HIV infection in situations where their husbands or sexual partners have sex with other partners. In this way, the HIV infection can be silently passed without a woman even knowing. This is often the case with casual sexual relationships or those involving migrant workers. Girls in such situations also tend to engage in sexual encounters at an earlier age than boys.

◆ In some African countries, many men leave their homes and loved ones and travel long distances to find work. In these areas the men seek out young women and teenage girls for sex and intimacy. The HIV infection rate among teenage girls and young adult women (20 – 25 year age group) is now very high. Many young teenage girls do not understand the serious HIV risk from having sex with older men.

Women are more vulnerable to HIV infection, and more easily infected than men.

The clinical course of HIV/AIDS in women

HIV infection and AIDS appear to run similar clinical courses in women as in men. However, women are vulnerable to specific gynaecological conditions, such as recurrent vaginal candida infection (thrush), genital herpes and cervical cancer *(see following pages)*.

The approach to treatment is generally the same as in men *(see Chapters 5 and 6)*. However, in women particular attention to reproductive tract infections is important. In addition, special consideration for pregnancy and contraception needs to be made *(see page 210)*.

In low socio-economic areas, the health status of women is often poor which makes women more susceptible to conditions such as anaemia, malnutrition, tuberculosis, gynaecological disorders, untreated or undetected sexually transmitted infections, urinary tract infections and disorders associated with pregnancy.

These and other conditions may lower a woman's health status even more and affect her immunity. This results in a more rapid progression towards HIV-related symptoms and AIDS than in a man.

◆ Detecting HIV infection in women

- ◆ Some women learn of their infection by voluntarily requesting an HIV test.

- ◆ Some women are detected HIV positive during medical investigation after developing symptoms of AIDS.

- ◆ However, most HIV-positive women find out:
  - – through routine antenatal screening
  - – while being treated for an STI
  - – after their sexual partner or newborn child is found to be HIV positive.

In these situations, the woman is often without any symptoms of HIV disease.

Providing sensitive counselling, education and information in these circumstances may influence her compliance with follow-up care and the adoption of safer sexual practices.

She may also need counselling and assistance in telling and dealing with her sexual partner.

It is vital that the proper counselling and preparation is provided to all women undergoing HIV tests, WHATEVER THE REASON FOR THE TEST. Informed consent for HIV testing is essential.

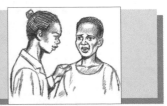

Genital tract infections in HIV-positive women

Genital tract infections in women are often more difficult to detect and to treat.

Candida albicans (thrush)

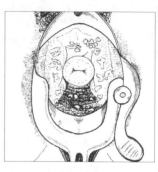

Vaginal thrush/candida

- This is commonly found in women with HIV infection and immune-deficiency.

- It presents with itching, discharge, white plaques and patches in the vagina, vulva and on the labia.

- There is often also candida infection in the mouth.

- It is most commonly seen when the CD4 count drops below 350 cells/mm³.

- The candida is often recurrent and may need longer therapy than usual, ongoing therapy or more powerful antifungal agents.

The treatment of vaginal candidiasis is discussed on page 136.

Sexually transmitted infections

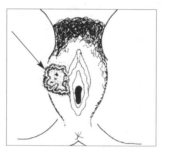

Chancroid ulcer

Other sexually transmitted infections, such as genital ulcer disease (syphilis, chancroid, herpes, lymphogranuloma, etc.), are common in women with HIV infection. Often the infection is more severe, unusual and more difficult to treat and cure.

Treatment may have to be for longer periods than normal and with more powerful or sophisticated drugs.

Chancroid infection

- This is often resistant to treatment and may be difficult to treat.
- It may persist for a long time.

The treatment of genital ulcer disease is discussed in Chapter 12.

Primary syphilis

- This should be treated as for secondary syphilis.

- Give benzathine penicillin injections 2,4 million units once a week for 3 weeks, to prevent the development of advanced disease or neuro-syphilis.

The treatment of primary syphilis is discussed in Chapter 12.

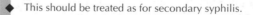

The effect of HIV on women's health

There is still a lot to learn about the natural effect of HIV infection on a woman's health. It appears that HIV does seem to have an influence on disease of the cervix and on genital tract infections.

Cervical disease and HIV infection

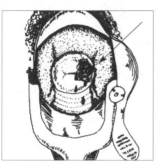

Cervical cancer

Some studies have shown that HIV infection may increase the risk of neoplasms (tumours) in the genital tract, especially carcinoma of the cervix. The risk may increase as the HIV disease gets worse. In addition, HIV may allow such neoplasms to progress at a faster rate than normal.

Cervicitis is also common in HIV-positive women.

PAP smears

For the reason above it is important to do a PAP smear of the cervix on all HIV-infected women every 1 – 2 years. It is important to stress the need for the woman to come back for the PAP smear result. Abnormal PAP smear results need to be managed actively to prevent the development of advanced cancer.

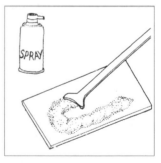

PAP smear

Women with abnormal smear results should be referred for gynaecological evaluation (colposcopy and biopsy) without delay. Follow-up of these results is essential.

> **A PAP smear should be done on all HIV-infected women every 1 – 2 years.**

Herpes genital infection

- This is often recurrent and may be more severe.

- It may reappear just before the menstrual period or during other illnesses.

- Pregnancy may also cause a recurrence of genital herpes.

- Occasionally regulating the menstrual periods with the oral contraceptive pill may help prevent the outbreak of menstrual-related genital herpes.

The treatment of herpes infection is discussed on pages 138 – 139.

Pelvic inflammatory disease (PID)

- This may be more severe in the presence of HIV infection.

- There is a tendency to develop abscesses with the need for surgical intervention.

The treatment of PID (vaginal discharge in women) is discussed on page 267.

Gonorrhoea and non-specific urethritis / cervicitis

- These may also be more severe with HIV infection.

The treatment of vaginal discharge and other STIs is discussed on pages 266 – 268.

> **Sexually transmitted infections may often be more severe, unusual and require longer treatment in women with HIV infection.**

Conditions in women commonly suggestive of immune-deficiency and advanced HIV disease (*see also page 103*)

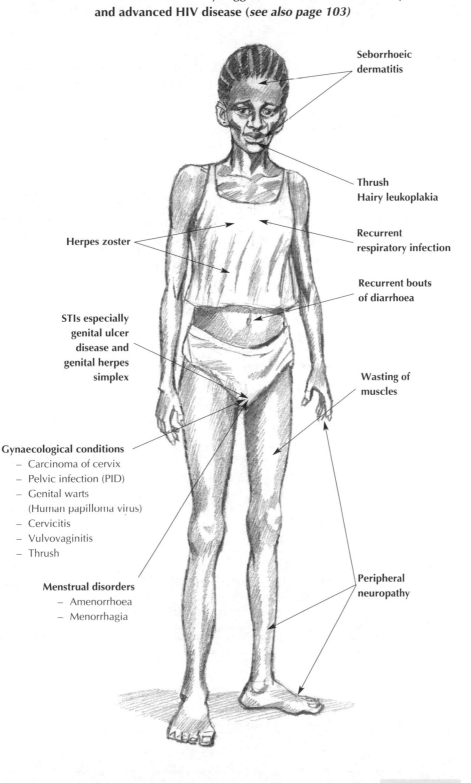

Seborrhoeic dermatitis

Thrush
Hairy leukoplakia

Recurrent respiratory infection

Recurrent bouts of diarrhoea

Herpes zoster

STIs especially genital ulcer disease and genital herpes simplex

Wasting of muscles

Gynaecological conditions
– Carcinoma of cervix
– Pelvic infection (PID)
– Genital warts
  (Human papilloma virus)
– Cervicitis
– Vulvovaginitis
– Thrush

Menstrual disorders
– Amenorrhoea
– Menorrhagia

Peripheral neuropathy

The effect of HIV on pregnancy and childbirth

Pregnancy is a very important and emotional period for a woman. There are many issues and considerations that HIV/AIDS presents to mothers, their partners, their families and to the health care workers during the pregnancy.

Pregnancy is often the first time a woman finds out that she is HIV positive. This may occur if an HIV test is part of the antenatal screening or if her newborn infant is found to have HIV/AIDS. This means that she now has to cope with the new crisis of an HIV diagnosis, and all the potential problems associated with this, as well as her pregnancy or newborn baby.

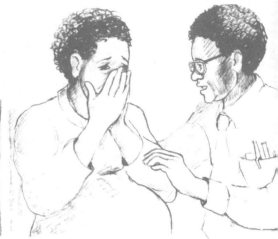

Pregnancy is an emotionally vulnerable and spiritual period. It is a time of life giving. To have to confront her own mortality, and to cope with a life-threatening disease during this time is extremely difficult for the mother. Often she may also have to deal with telling her partner as well. He may also be HIV positive or he may react very badly or aggressively to the news.

In some women with advanced HIV disease, the possibility of dying soon, or not long after the birth of the baby, may be a very real possibility.

The International Planned Parenthood Federation has stressed that HIV-infected women have the right to exercise their reproductive choice.

◆ The effects of pregnancy and HIV infection

AIDS and pregnancy raise many important considerations.

The effect of pregnancy on the HIV disease

Pregnancy **does not** seem to have any significant effect on the progress
of HIV disease in the **early asymptomatic phase**.

Pregnancy may affect women who have more advanced HIV disease and cause
the disease to progress more rapidly to AIDS.

The effect of HIV disease on pregnancy

HIV infection does not usually appear to seriously affect the pregnancy.
However, reports from parts of Africa do suggest that HIV infection may cause
an increased likelihood of intra-uterine growth retardation, prematurity, still-births
and congenital infections.

ARV drug toxicity may occur and complicate pregnancy. Recent reports of fatal lactic
acidosis in pregnant women on DDI and d4T suggest these drugs should be avoided
in pregnancy.

HIV infection of the foetus / newborn

An HIV positive woman has approximately a 30% chance of transmitting the HIV
virus to her infant. This may occur during pregnancy, childbirth and also during
breast feeding.

Several factors have been identified which may help to predict when a mother
may pass the virus on to the foetus during pregnancy or during breast feeding.

These factors include the following:

- The stage of disease – there is more likelihood of passing the infection
  on if the mother has the symptomatic / advanced stage of disease.

- A high HIV viral load in the mother will increase the risk for mother to child
  transmission (MTCT).

- A low CD4 count.

- The time of infection – if the mother acquires new HIV infection just before
  the pregnancy, during the pregnancy or while breast feeding.

- Obstetric factors and other factors *(see Chapter 10)*

- There are many strategies in pregnancy, childbirth and infant feeding that can
  reduce the chance of MTCT. *These are discussed in Chapter 10.*

WOMEN WITH HIV/AIDS

◆ HIV screening during pregnancy

HIV screening during pregnancy
needs careful and sensitive consideration ▬▬▬▬▬▬▬▬▬▬▬

There are many advantages of knowing whether a woman is HIV positive during her pregnancy.

◆ The woman can be offered ART if necessary (*see Chapter 5*).

◆ She can be counselled and informed about the risks of MTCT and ways to prevent the MTCT.

◆ She can be counselled and informed about a termination of pregnancy so that she can make informed decisions whether to continue the pregnancy or not.

◆ Her partner / spouse may also be infected. This is important as she may need further counselling about how to tell her partner etc.

◆ Her newborn infant will need to be followed up and monitored for HIV infection.

The importance of voluntary testing
and counselling of pregnant women ▬▬▬▬▬▬▬▬▬▬▬

◆ New developments in HIV/AIDS and increased knowledge about various aspects of transmission and prevention have increased the options available to patients and mothers with HIV/AIDS.

◆ These new developments may influence a woman's decision:
  – to become pregnant;
  – to continue with her pregnancy;
  – to consider various options for preventing mother to child transmission;
  – to access anti-retroviral therapy.

◆ In many situations it is now very important and advantageous for the expectant mother to know her HIV status. There are many important issues surrounding HIV testing and how individuals cope with a HIV positive test result.

◆ Issues of stigma and discrimination are also major problems experienced by people with HIV/AIDS. It may also be a disadvantage for only the woman to be tested as this may result in undue blame and other negative consequences.

◆ Ideally the woman and her partner should be tested at the same time. This promotes joint responsibility and decision-making regarding sexual practices, reproduction, maternal care and infant care.

◆ Involuntary testing of a woman during her pregnancy, or testing without informed consent, is a violation of rights and is not acceptable.

◆ Counselling and testing should only be done on a voluntary basis, with informed consent. It must be carried out in privacy and the results must be dealt with in a confidential manner.

◆ If testing is carried out, then the woman needs to be told about:
  – the benefits of testing;
  – and how the test may influence various therapeutic and other options.

◆ The primary purpose of counselling and testing is to encourage informed decision-making and behaviour. It is therefore very important for individuals to have access to the necessary services they need e.g.
  – ART (if available)
  – family planning (to avoid pregnancy)
  – condoms to practice safer sex during pregnancy and breast feeding
  – primary care services for HIV care for adults and children
  – ongoing counselling services for individuals needing further support
  – prevention of mother to child transmission (MTCT)

◆ It is recognised that many services operate under difficult conditions with major deficiencies. HIV testing must always be very carefully considered, especially where services are basic and unable to provide acceptable support for HIV-positive mothers and their partners.

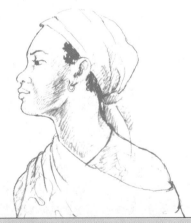

A decision to screen a woman for HIV infection is a joint consideration between the health worker and the woman but the *final* decision should be made by the woman herself.

Any HIV testing must be accompanied by careful and adequate pre-test counselling with proper post-test counselling and support.

Confidentiality of the result is important.

WOMEN WITH HIV/AIDS

◆ Care during pregnancy and childbirth

As described on *page 205*, pregnancy is often the time when a woman finds out that she has HIV/AIDS. It is also a very special time and HIV infection has many medical, psychological and social implications for the mother and her family.

Women are often willing to adopt healthier lifestyle changes during pregnancy. These may include diet, rest, avoidance of smoking, alcohol and drugs, regular health checks etc. Also it is a good time to educate women (and their partners) about safer sexual practices, contraception and about AIDS in general.

The health care services and the health workers should make a great effort to establish good support and care structures to manage women, their partners and their newborn. Support and care will need to be considered for the family. Occasionally, with a very ill mother, care arrangements may have to be made for the newborn or for other children in the family.

Ideally the health service should try to provide a team comprising doctors, midwives, counsellors, educators and social workers for the care of HIV-infected women.

Many women who are pregnant and HIV-infected are from lower socio-economic backgrounds and are already suffering from socio-economic hardships. HIV infection, and its effects, add considerably to this burden.

Antenatal care

Extra antenatal care and attention

◆ Women with HIV infection need extra care during pregnancy. They should be seen more frequently than usual.

◆ Invasive diagnostic procedures, such as chorionic villus sampling and amniocentesis, should be avoided unless absolutely necessary.

◆ It is important to keep a look-out for the development of any HIV-related conditions (*see Chapter 7*) and especially for infections, such as vaginal and oral thrush, and other opportunistic infections, such as herpes.

◆ The HIV condition is monitored and managed as usual during the pregnancy. The CD4 count may not be very stable and constant during pregnancy. The CD4 count is 25% lower in pregnancy and the CD4 percentage is unchanged. CD4 counts return to pre-pregnancy levels approximately 3 months after delivery. This may mean that the levels need to be repeated on a few occasions if the CD4 count is to be used for making important management decisions e.g. for prophylaxis of opportunistic infections etc.

Anti-retroviral therapy (ART) during pregnancy

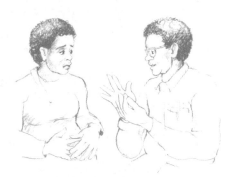

◆ Women already on ART should generally continue during pregnancy. Some clinicians interrupt the therapy for the first trimester (14 weeks) of pregnancy and continue it from the second trimester onwards. Any ARVs that may harm the foetus should be discontinued and substituted e.g. efavirenz, hydroxyurea.

◆ If a woman is found to require ART during her pregnancy it is best if the ART is given from the second trimester onwards with 'pregnancy friendly' ARVs.

◆ AZT, 3TC and nevirapine may be used as there is much more experience with these drugs in pregnancy. Protease inhibitors can also be used. Their side effects, however, need to be considered (especially indinavir – renal calculi and hyperbilirubinaemia).

◆ Efavirenz and hydroxyurea are harmful to the foetus and should not be given during pregnancy.

◆ ddI (and ddC) in combination with d4T should also be avoided due to potential lactic acidosis in the mother.

◆ ART recommendations during pregnancy are provided on *pages 231 – 232*.

The specific ARV agents and regimens used for the prevention of MTCT in pregnancy are discussed in Chapter 10.

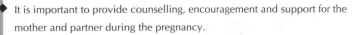

'Pregnancy friendly' anti-retrovirals are preferred for pregnant mothers.
See also Chapter 10, pages 231 – 232

Emotional support

◆ It is important to provide counselling, encouragement and support for the mother and partner during the pregnancy.

◆ It is also important to start preparing the mother for possible problems that may occur after the pregnancy (breast/bottle feeding, follow-up and HIV diagnosis in the newborn, a treatment and care programme etc.).

WOMEN WITH HIV/AIDS

Childbirth / labour

◆ ART should be given to the mother to help prevent MTCT *(see Chapter 10)*.

◆ Every effort should be made to avoid even minor trauma to the baby during birth as this may promote transmission of the virus to the baby.

◆ Avoid artificial rupture of membranes and especially prolonged rupture of membranes.

◆ Elective Caesarean section has been shown to reduce the risk of MTCT (if viral load is > 1 000).

◆ Avoid prolonged labour.

◆ Health workers should avoid using procedures such as foetal scalp monitoring, forceps delivery and vacuum extraction, if possible, as these may cause minor skin lacerations and abrasions.

◆ All injection sites on newborn babies must be properly cleaned before inserting the needle, to make sure the mother's blood is not on the skin.

Health workers must be adequately protected during childbirth. Ideally gloves, aprons, gowns and eye protectors should be worn.

Strategies to prevent mother to child transmission during pregnancy are discussed in Chapter 10.

Post-partum

◆ The mother should breast feed her infant exclusively for up to 6 months, switching completely to replacement feeding when it is safe to do so. Feeding of infants of HIV-positive mothers is discussed in *Chapter 10*.

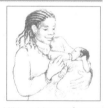

HIV-positive mothers can use formula feed if it can be done adequately and safely

◆ Give the infant ARV prophylaxis for at least 6 weeks after birth *(see Chapter 10)*.

◆ Bromocriptine (Parlodel) 2,5 mg orally 12 hourly for 14 days or 1 ampoule Parlodel LA IMI stat can be used to stop lactation if necessary.

◆ An HIV PCR test could be done on the newborn after 4 weeks if ART is available *(see page 40)*.

◆ BCG immunisation should be given to newborns as usual, unless the infant is very ill *(also see page 200)*.

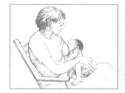

HIV-positive mothers are advised to breast feed exclusively if infant formula feeding cannot be given safely and adequately

◆ The usual post-partum care should be given to the mother.

Ways to prevent MTCT during pregnancy, childbirth and breast feeding are discussed in detail in Chapter 10.

◆ Continuing or terminating the pregnancy?

In some countries, termination of pregnancy may be considered as there is a very real risk of transmitting the HIV infection to the foetus. Good ART care and delivery can however significantly reduce the risk of MTCT.

The desire to conceive and produce a healthy child is often overwhelming. Mothers (and their partners) need to be carefully counselled. The risks and chances of transmission need to be carefully and sensitively explained. Strategies to prevent MTCT can be very successful *(see Chapter 10)*.

Parents must make their own decisions and choices.

The possibility of transmitting the infection to the foetus will raise many other problems and considerations for the mother and her partner. These include the following:

◆ Understanding the risk and the available options to reduce the risk of MTCT *(see Chapter 10)*

◆ The choice of a termination of the pregnancy

◆ The difficulties of diagnosing HIV infection in newborns

◆ The possibility of caring for a sick and dying infant

◆ The possible feelings of guilt, sadness and fear

If the HIV infection is newly diagnosed:

◆ The mother will need to deal with changing her sexual practices (towards safer sex). This may cause problems *(see page 287)*.

◆ The HIV infection may also require special care during the pregnancy, labour and postnatally (infant feeding).

◆ There will need to be special considerations for infant feeding.

◆ She will have to consider possible prevention of future pregnancies.

◆ There may be a possibility of one or both parents dying while the child is still young.

◆ Often the woman is already suffering with low socio-economic hardships, and having HIV infection can severely increase the burden.

HIV and pregnancy demand very special attention and sensitivity. Women (and their partners) need careful counselling, support and encouragement during this period.

WOMEN WITH HIV/AIDS

Contraception for women with HIV infection

It is important for HIV-infected women to be properly informed about the risks of transmitting HIV to their foetuses during pregnancy and childbirth. They will then be able to make any final decisions for themselves about whether to have children or not.

Most contraceptives can be used in women who have HIV infection i.e. condoms, combined oral contraceptive pills, progesterone-only pills, injectable progesterones, spermicidals and sterilization. Some are more reliable than others.

The intra-uterine device is not recommended.

Condoms

◆ Condoms are an ideal form of contraception as they are the only contraceptive which also helps prevent the transmission of HIV during sexual intercourse.

◆ All other contraceptives do not prevent the spread of HIV. An HIV-positive woman, who does not use condoms for contraception, must understand that her partner is at high risk of acquiring HIV from her. Also it is important to prevent getting re-infected with HIV as this can advance the progression of the HIV disease more rapidly.

◆ Other forms of contraception will not protect a woman from acquiring HIV from an HIV-positive man.

◆ When condoms are used properly they can provide a reasonably reliable form of contraception and there is only a small pregnancy failure rate.

◆ Female condoms are becoming more easily available.

Intra-uterine contraceptive device (IUCD)

◆ These are not generally recommended as they may promote pelvic inflammatory disease (PID) in the woman. This may also increase her chance of spreading the HIV to her male partner.

◆ The string or tail of the IUCD may cause minor abrasions to her partner's penis and this may aid HIV transmission to her partner.

◆ IUCDs may also increase menstrual blood flow and the chance of HIV transmission.

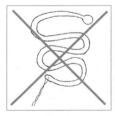

Intra-uterine contraceptive device (IUCD)

Oral contraceptives

◆ These can be safely and reliably used. They may, however, change the integrity of the genital tract and make the women more susceptible to HIV infection.

◆ Some of the oral contraceptives may alter the metabolism of certain drugs
  – some drugs, such as rifampicin and tetracyclines, may also interfere with the oral contraceptive and result in contraceptive failure.

◆ Some ART drugs (PIs and NNRTIs) may interfere with oral contraceptives, reducing their effectiveness. Clinicians should check this with the inserts in the drug packages. A higher dose (50 mg) of oestrogen component should be used.

◆ Long-acting injectable progestagens may alter the mucous in the cervical canal. This may affect other parts of the genital tract as well. Studies are currently being done to find out if these changes have any influence on the transmission of HIV.

Spermicidal preparations

◆ Some spermicidal preparations which contain nonoxynol-9 may inhibit the HIV virus. This may assist in the prevention of HIV transmission. However, the effectiveness is not yet clear, and this cannot be regarded as a safe method of preventing HIV transmission.

◆ The use of condoms is much more effective in combination with a spermicidal preparation.

> **Condoms are the only contraceptive that can reliably prevent HIV spreading from one partner to another.**

Prophylaxis after sexual exposure

◆ ART can help prevent HIV infection after sexual abuse / rape

This is especially necessary in the following situations:

◆ When rape has occured

◆ If the condom slips off during sex with an HIV-positive person

◆ In other situations when unwanted or risky sex has occurred

HIV prophylaxis after sexual exposure includes:

◆ Gently cleansing the genital area

◆ Administration of ART. This medication should be started as early as possible, and preferably within the first 2 – 3 hours of the sexual exposure. Guidelines for this therapy follow the same approach as prophylaxis after needlestick injuries *(see pages 322 – 323)*. The therapy should be continued for 4 weeks.

General recommendations:

◆ If possible the HIV status of the source person (i.e. the rapist, sexual partner etc.) should be determined as soon as possible *(see page 321)*.

◆ HIV-antibody tests should be performed at 6 weeks, 3 months and 6 months in order to determine whether HIV infection occurred.

◆ Alternatively, an HIV PCR test can be done approximately 10 days after exposure.

◆ Counselling should be provided, especially after rape.

Prophylaxis after sexual exposure should only be offered in situations of rape, unwanted sex or very risky sexual events. It should not become a habit or used routinely or frequently in place of general safer sexual practice.

Counselling of people with HIV and AIDS is discussed in detail in Chapter 13.
The prevention of MTCT is discussed in Chapter 10.

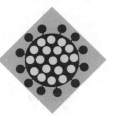

Chapter 10

REDUCING MOTHER TO CHILD HIV TRANSMISSION

General introduction

Mother to child is a well-established mode of HIV transmission. Infection may occur during pregnancy, during the labour or from breast feeding. Approximately 25 – 30% of HIV-infected mothers will transmit the HIV infection to their infants, and 70 – 75% of infants will **not** contract HIV from their HIV-positive mothers.

> **Mother to child HIV transmission can take place during pregnancy, childbirth or breast feeding.**

Mother to child HIV transmission (MTCT) during pregnancy and labour

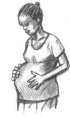

The following section deals with a practical approach for reducing vertical HIV transmission during pregnancy and labour. Various recommendations are made, some of which may not be affordable for some patients, e.g. the section on ART. Health care workers will need to treat patients in the most appropriate way for their situation.

There are numerous ways to prevent the transmission of HIV from mother to child during pregnancy and childbirth. These ways can be implemented in the **antenatal and labour phases of the pregnancy, and post delivery.**

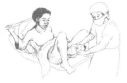

Mother to child transmission during infant feeding is dealt with on page 233.

◆ Risk factors for mother to child HIV transmission

The following factors are likely to increase the risk of MTCT:

HIV viral load

- The higher the viral load, especially greater than 100 000 copies / mm^3, the more likelihood that MTCT will occur.

- Women with advanced HIV disease (AIDS), are likely to have a high viral load.

- Any situation which may result in a high load, or even a brief increase in load, will add to the risk e.g. infection episodes such as tuberculosis, or a newly acquired HIV infection.

- Different HIV viral types and characteristics can also influence the risk.

- Women with very low viral loads (< 1 000) have a very low likelihood of MTCT.

Immune status

- The risk for MTCT is increased the more severe the immune-deficiency.

- This is probably because of the relationship between immune-deficiency and viral load.

- Women with low CD4 counts (< 200 cells / mm^3 or < 15%) are more likely to transmit HIV to their infants.

Clinical state of the mother

- Mothers with advanced disease or AIDS are more likely to transmit HIV than mothers in the earlier or asymptomatic phase of the disease.

- This feature is most likely associated with higher viral loads and low CD4 cell counts.

Placental infection (chorio-amnionitis)

- Infection of the chorion or the amnion may increase the chance of MTCT.

- Genital infections, and especially sexually transmitted infections (STIs), may result in chorio-amnionitis.

- Prolonged rupture of membranes during labour is another common cause of placental infection.

Foetal trauma

- Traumatic births, and births where the foetal skin is traumatised from obstetrical procedures, increase the risk of MTCT.

- A Caesarean section may offer some protection against MTCT as it is less traumatic on the baby than most vaginal births.

Vitamin A deficiency

- Studies have shown that there is an association between Vitamin A deficiency in the mother and risk of MTCT.

Prematurity

- Any pre-term birth or low birth weight will place a baby at higher risk for MTCT.

Maternal breast conditions

- Mastitis, breast abscesses or other inflammatory breast conditions can increase the risk of MTCT.

New HIV infections

- Newly acquired HIV infection just prior to, or during, pregnancy or breast feeding increases the risk of MTCT.

Prevention of MTCT during the ANTENATAL period

Prevention of any new HIV infection

◆ Any new HIV infection during pregnancy and breast feeding is likely to result in an increase in the HIV viraemia. This is considered to increase the likelihood of MTCT.

◆ For this reason pregnant mothers must be informed of this risk and educated on safer sexual practices. It is especially important for them to use condoms if their partner is HIV-infected, or if his HIV status is unknown.

N.B. The above also applies to a woman who is already known to be HIV positive. This is because new additional HIV infections may add new strains, and / or result in a transient increased HIV viraemia (*see page 76*).

Preventing new HIV infections during pregnancy will help reduce MTCT.

Prevention and treatment of sexually transmitted infections (STIs)

◆ Effective prevention and treatment of any STI and of any other genital infection will:
  – reduce the likelihood of placental infection (chorio-amnionitis) and reduce the risk of MTCT
  – a pap smear should be done

Multivitamins

◆ Nutritional supplements (iron and folate) are often routinely given during pregnancy.

◆ Multivitamins, including Vitamin A, should be further supplemented, especially in mothers from lower socio-economic groups where undernutrition is common.

◆ Multivitamin supplements should be given from the initial booking, or diagnosis of pregnancy, until delivery. This may help to prevent premature birth, and may therefore reduce the risk of MTCT.

Anti-retroviral therapy (ART) prophylaxis

ART prophylaxis should be considered for known HIV-positive women. It is now well established that ART prophylaxis during pregnancy and labour can reduce MTCT by 50 – 60%. If resources permit, then ART prophylaxis is recommended for HIV-positive women. Regimens for ART may change rapidly, and readers should keep themselves informed of these changes (*see the following pages*).

Clinic visits and assessment

◆ During the antenatal visits, pregnant HIV-positive mothers should be carefully assessed. Look at their risk for further HIV infection and do a PAP smear.

◆ The HIV disease should be assessed by clinically looking for signs of HIV infection and immune deficiency *(see Chapters 3, 5 and 6)*. A viral load and CD4 cell count should be done if possible. The HIV disease may need treatment *(see pages 231 – 232 for use of ART during pregnancy)*.

◆ Prophylaxis for opportunistic infections i.e. co-trimoxazole can be given from the second trimester onwards if necessary. Pregnant mothers should not be vaccinated.

Follow-up visits

These should occur monthly until 28 weeks, 2-weekly until 36 weeks, then weekly unless more frequent visits are needed for health or obstetric reasons.

Foetal monitoring

◆ Non-invasive foetal monitoring such as ultrasounds should be done as usual. Special attention is needed in mothers with CD4 cell counts < 200 or with other adverse conditions such as illness, substance abuse etc. This will help to prevent pre-term labour and low birth weight.

Laboratory tests

The following tests should be done if possible:

◆ Full blood count at first visit and again at 6 months if all is well

◆ CD4 cell count at first visit and at 6 months

◆ Hepatitis B and C serology at first visit and at 6 months if all is well

◆ Blood group, Rh screen, rubella titre, RPR / VDRL

◆ HIV viral load at first visit and at 36 weeks

◆ STI screen at first visit; vaginal wet preparation, gonococcus, bacterial vaginosis, chlamydia repeated at 32 – 36 weeks

Avoid invasive procedures

◆ Amniocentesis, chorion villus sampling and cordocentesis and external cephalic version should be avoided as these procedures can increase risk for MTCT.

Counselling sexual practice

◆ Counselling for safe sexual practice during pregnancy is very important. Try to include the sexual partner in the counselling if possible.

Provide ART

◆ *See pages 231 – 232* for the provision of ART during pregnancy

Prevention of MTCT during the CHILDBIRTH period (labour / intrapartum)

There are various ways to reduce the chances of MTCT during labour:

Provide ART

If resources are available, it is best to provide ART during labour *(see pages 231 – 232)*.

Method of delivery

◆ Ensure mother has taken ARV medication *(see page 231)*.

◆ Normal vaginal delivery is recommended unless viral load is very high. Prophylactic antibiotics are not recommended for normal vaginal births.

◆ Caesarean section has been shown to reduce the risk of MTCT. However, it is not routinely indicated in HIV-positive mothers because it has other potential risks. It is also costly.

◆ Caesarean section should be done in women with very high viral loads and if there is any obstetric indication. Prolonged or obstructed labour should be avoided.

◆ Prophylactic antibiotics should be given for all Caesarean deliveries in HIV-positive mothers.

◆ Delivery staff must adhere to universal precautions, including eye protection, to prevent contamination with the mother's blood and body fluids etc.

Vaginal cleansing

Some studies have shown that vaginal cleansing with an antiseptic solution may have some benefit by reducing vertical HIV transmission.

See the following page for more information.

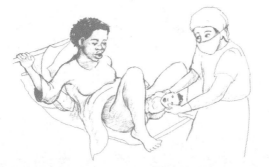

℞

Vaginal cleansing

◆ The vaginal canal is cleansed with 0,25% chlorhexidene solution during vaginal examinations

– the solution is made by adding 12,5 ml chlorhexidene to 5 litres of water.

Technique

Before vaginal examination in labour, the vulval area must be cleaned with the solution as follows:

◆ Sterile gloves must be worn.

◆ Wrap a thick or double gauze swab around the two examining finger tips

– pinch the free edges securely between the two fingers.

◆ Soak the swabs with the chlorhexidene solution in a galley pot

– or pour the solution over swabs.

– or spray the swabs very well using a swab bottle.

◆ Open the vulvae with the left hand and carefully clean the whole vaginal surface with the soaked swabs.

◆ Discard the swabs and keep the vulval area open while inserting examining fingers, preferably using chlorhexidene obstetric cream.

Avoid artificial rupture of membranes (AROM)

◆ Ruptured membranes for longer than 4 hours prior to delivery is associated with increased transmission of HIV from mother to child.

◆ There is no clinically important benefit to do *routine* ROM, in any pregnancy, in HIV-positive or -negative women.

However in HIV-positive pregnancies, AROM should be avoided if at all possible. This will help to reduce HIV MTCT.

◆ AROM should only be done

– if there are specific obstetric indications

– as late as possible.

In HIV-positive women other methods of progressing labour should be considered, e.g. oxytocin augmentation or possibly Caesarean section if indicated.

Uses of AROM and recommendations to prevent HIV MTCT	
Use of AROM	Recommendation/modification
Poor progress of labour	Oxytocin augmentation or Caesarean section
Diagnosis of meconium-stained liquor (MSL) as an indicator of foetal distress	AROM is an inaccurate marker of foetal distress and should not be used for this purpose alone.
For diagnosis of meconium-stained liquor, to enable suctioning of the newborn's airway	AROM should only be done for this purpose during the second stage of labour, just before suctioning is required.
For internal foetal monitoring	Only if foetal distress is suspected and external monitoring is unsuccessful. The risk and benefits from this procedure must be carefully considered in each case. In HIV-positive women internal monitoring should be avoided if possible.
For amnio-infusion	The benefits and risks must be considered in each case.

Avoid trauma to the foetus

◆ Any trauma to the foetal head or other body parts should be avoided as much as possible.

◆ The following may result in trauma and must be avoided if possible:
  − needle-type foetal scalp electrodes
  − instrument deliveries
  − over-vigorous suctioning of the infant

Avoid episiotomies

◆ Episiotomy may increase the risk of MTCT by increased exposure of the foetus to maternal blood.

◆ There are very few clinical benefits for routine episiotomy.

◆ Avoid episiotomy except for:
  − prolonged second stage
  − foetal distress
  − medical indications to shorten second stage

◆ Often delivery can be helped by an upright posture (e.g. crouching / squatting) and by encouraging the patient to bear down.

Prevention of MTCT AFTER the BIRTH
(post partum) – management of the newborn

Avoidance of trauma to the newborn

Care must be taken not to traumatise the newborn after birth. The mother's body fluids must be removed from the newborn.

The following is recommended for all births including Caesarean section:

◆ Gently wipe away secretions from the newborn's face with a soft towel or tissue.

◆ Avoid unnecessary suctioning which may cause trauma to mucous membranes, and may facilitate the passage of viral infection.

◆ In most births suctioning is totally unnecessary. It is indicated if there is thick fluid in the newborn's airway such as meconium-stained liquor or excessive fluids.

◆ Give the newborn baby ARV prophylaxis medication for the first 6 weeks of life as outlined on *pages 231 – 232*.

◆ If possible, the newborn should be breast fed. Formula feeding can be considered where this is safe. *Pages 233 – 240 deal with the issue of baby feeding in detail.*

Anti-retroviral therapy (ART) to prevent MTCT

ART is the most important strategy to prevent MTCT. HIV-positive mothers should be given ART during pregnancy and childbirth, and the newborn should be given 6 weeks of ART as prophylaxis (prevention). ART should also be considered for HIV-positive mothers who are breast feeding.

There is no single regimen that is preferred. Research is ongoing to determine which regimen is most appropriate for various clinical situations.

The following are important considerations:

◆ The affordability of the medication

◆ The possibility of developing HIV drug resistance in the mother which may affect her future options for HIV care (especially with nevirapine use)

◆ Whether the mother has drug-resistant HIV virus (from previously failed ART)

◆ The level of HIV viral load in the mother

> **It is critical that as many HIV-positive women as possible access MTCT ART. Antenatal clinics need to improve HIV testing and counselling services in order to achieve success in MTCT prevention programmes.**

℞

HIV-positive women who are pregnant and are already on ART

During pregnancy

◆ ART safety in the first 14 weeks of pregnancy is not fully established. It is safest to discontinue the medication during the first trimester of pregnancy. All ARV medication should be discontinued and restarted from about 12 – 14 weeks of pregnancy.

◆ AZT has the most well-known safety profile in pregnancy and should usually form part of a pregnancy regimen. AZT should never be used with d4T. Nevirapine and 3TC have also been widely used in pregnancy and are considered to be relatively safe in pregnancy.

◆ ddI / ddC and d4T combinations during pregnancy are not safe and should not be used in pregnancy. If the mother is on these drugs they should be stopped and alternative drugs used.

◆ Efivirenz should not be used in pregnancy and should be replaced with another appropriate drug.

During labour

Whatever the ARV regimen the following should apply during labour:

◆ AZT intravenously 2 mg / kg infusion for the first hour, then 1 mg / kg hourly by continuous infusion until delivery.

Newborn ARV prophylaxis for 6 weeks

◆ AZT 2 mg / kg every 6 hours for 6 weeks or 0,4 ml / kg 12 hourly

---

℞

ART for HIV-positive pregnant women who present within the first 34 weeks of pregnancy and who have not previously been on ART

During pregnancy

◆ Commence AZT as early as possible after 14 weeks (200 – 300 mg 12 hourly).

◆ 3TC 150 mg 12 hourly can also be added if affordable.

◆ Use nevirapine 200 mg 12 hourly (daily for the first 14 days) especially if viral load is high and CD4 cell count is low.

During labour

◆ Give AZT intravenously 2 mg / kg infusion for the first hour, then 1 mg / kg hourly by continuous infusion until delivery.

Newborn ARV prophylaxis for 6 weeks

◆ Treat with AZT 2 mg / kg every 6 hours or 0,4 ml / kg 12 hourly.

◆ 3TC 0,2 ml / kg 12 hourly can also be given.

◆ Nevirapine 2 mg / kg within 72 hours of birth can also be given.

℞

ART for HIV-positive pregnant women who present after 34 weeks of pregnancy who have not previously been on ART

During last 4 – 6 weeks of pregnancy

◆ Commence AZT 200 – 300 mg 12 hourly.

◆ 3TC 150 mg 12 hourly can also be added if affordable.

During labour

◆ Give AZT intravenously 2 mg / kg infusion for the first hour, then 1 mg / kg hourly by continuous infusion until delivery.

◆ Nevirapine 200 mg orally can also be given.

Newborn ARV prophylaxis for 6 weeks

◆ Treat with AZT 2 mg / kg every 6 hours or 0,4 ml / kg 12 hourly.

◆ 3TC 0,2 ml / kg 12 hourly can also be given if affordable.

◆ Nevirapine 2 mg / kg within 72 hours of birth can also be given.

℞

ART for HIV-positive pregnant women who present in labour or who have not received any antenatal ART

◆ Treat with single-dose nevirapine 200 mg orally at the onset of labour or as soon thereafter as possible.

Newborn prophylaxis

◆ Treat with nevirapine 2 mg / kg orally at 48 – 72 hours.

◆ AZT 2 mg / kg every 6 hours or 0.4 ml / kg 12 hourly and 3TC 0,2 ml / kg 12 hourly can also be given if affordable. Use for 1 week and extend to 6 weeks if affordable.

℞

If the mother is only diagnosed HIV positive after birth

◆ Give AZT 2 mg / kg every 6 hours or 0,4 ml / kg 12 hourly for 6 weeks if affordable.

Adapted from: Gray GE, McIntyre JA, Jivkov B, Violari A, 'Preventing mother to child transmission of HIV-1 in South Africa.' Southern African Journal of HIV Medicine, Issue 4: 15-26

Prevention of MTCT during INFANT FEEDING

◆ Mother to child HIV transmission (MTCT) during breast feeding

HIV can be transmitted from mother to child during pregnancy, during childbirth itself and through breast feeding. *MTCT prevention during pregnancy and labour is discussed on pages 212 – 232.* This section deals with the feeding of babies of HIV-positive mothers in general and in particular how to reduce the risk of transmission during feeding.

(This section has been written after consultation and in accord with WHO, UNAIDS and UNICEF guidelines.)

◆ Points to note

◆ The majority of babies who are breast fed by HIV-infected mothers are not infected.

◆ The risk of the baby being infected is greater if the mother acquires the HIV infection while she is breast feeding or if she is re-infected during breast feeding.

◆ For most babies born in Africa, the risk of death through not being breast fed through the first few months of life is greater than the risk of being infected with HIV.

◆ Because conditions in many parts of Africa make other methods of feeding dangerous, most HIV-infected mothers will breast feed their babies.

◆ Calculating the risks of MTCT

◆ It is estimated that the baby of a HIV mother has a 15 – 30% chance of being infected during pregnancy and delivery.

◆ The baby of an HIV-infected mother who is breast fed for 24 months has an additional 10 – 20% chance of being infected through breast milk.

◆ This risk can be reduced by exclusive breast feeding for 6 months, good breast feeding technique, and the avoidance of further HIV infection in the mother. If it is safe to do so, breast feeding should cease at 6 months, and other feeding methods used thereafter.

> **Health workers need to do all they can to support the HIV-infected mother who breast feeds during the first few months of the infant's life. The mother will need both practical and emotional support.**

Some definitions

Replacement feeding: The WHO definition is 'the process of feeding a child who is not receiving any breast milk with a diet that provides all the nutrients a child needs until the child is fully fed on family foods'.

Complementary feeding: when a child is receiving other foods as well as breast milk or breast milk substitute.

Exclusive breast feeding: when a baby receives only breast milk (no water or any other fluid).

◆ Factors affecting MTCT during breast feeding

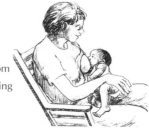

◆ HIV-infected 'immune cells' are present in the breast milk of HIV-positive mothers. These infected cells are found in the breast milk throughout the breast feeding period. MTCT from breast feeding can therefore occur any time during the feeding. Breast milk also contains anti-infective factors which help the baby fight HIV.

◆ MTCT during breast feeding is more likely:

– if the mother contracts a new HIV infection during breast feeding

– if there are clinical signs of AIDS in the mother (*see Chapter 6*)

– where laboratory tests show the mother has a high HIV viral load or a low CD4 cell count (*see pages 73 – 74*). In rural areas it may not be possible to monitor these factors.

The following factors may also affect MTCT:

◆ Breast conditions, such as sore nipples and mastitis. This is often the result of poor breast feeding management such as poor attachment, delayed and restricted breast feeding after the birth, and mixed feeding.

◆ Thrush in mother and/or baby. This is usually present in both mother and baby. It is a serious complication for breast feeding and may be triggered by the prescription of antibiotics to mother or baby, or due to immune deficiency in the mother.

◆ Choice of infant feeding

From birth to 6 months

Milk in some form is essential. The options include:

◆ Exclusive breast feeding, that is feeding with breast milk **only**, by the mother or another woman (wet nurse) who is HIV negative.

◆ Expressed breast milk, whether from the mother or from a well-regulated milk bank where donated milk is heated to remove HIV.

◆ Commercial infant formula – this meets the nutritional needs of the baby for the first 6 months of life but it does not contain any immune protective factors, which can prevent many infections.

◆ Home-prepared formula which can be prepared from fresh cows', goats' or sheep's milk. Cows' milk can be modified for babies by mixing 50 ml of water for each 100 ml of milk, and adding 10 g of sugar. However, these formulas do not provide the micronutrients the baby needs, especially iron, zinc and Vitamins A and C and foliate. Micronutrient supplements have to be added to home-prepared formula.

◆ Powdered full-cream milk and evaporated milks. These can be modified in a similar way to fresh milk (*see above*). Addition of micronutrients is needed.

◆ **There is a high risk that replacement feeding may place the baby at risk from infectious diseases such as gastro-enteritis and respiratory infections, which can lead to malnutrition. According to a WHO review of available evidence in 1999, infants who are not breast fed are 6 times more likely to die.**

◆ **Recent research suggests that the mixed feeding of infants, traditional in many parts of Africa, carries a greater risk of MTCT than exclusive breast feeding. This is when breast milk is complemented with other foods from an early age.**

From 6 months to 2 years

From six months a baby needs to start eating nutritious solid food as well as having milk. When the mother is HIV infected, one way of reducing the risk of MTCT is to stop breast feeding when complementary feeding is started.

◆ Feeding with milk should continue after 6 months. This can be with a commercially manufactured formula or with home-prepared formula. When these are not available, fresh cows' milk may be adequate, provided the baby is receiving sufficient nutrients from the remainder of his or her diet.

◆ Complementary foods made properly from nutritionally enriched family foods should be given three times a day.

◆ If possible other animal products, such as meat, fish and eggs, should be given as a source of iron, protein, vitamins and zinc.

◆ If possible other milk products, such as unmodified animal milk, dried skimmed milk and yoghurt should be included as a source of protein and calcium.

◆ Legume-based foods, for example mashed beans, peas, peanut butter or soya products, are relatively high in protein.

◆ Fruit and vegetables provide vitamins, especially A and C.

Most HIV-infected mothers in Africa will have to breast feed their babies. The best way to reduce the chances of MTCT is by helping the mother breast feed her baby exclusively for up to 6 months, and then to support her in the change to replacement feeding.

◆ ART and MTCT

If ART is available and affordable and if it can be offered on a sustainable basis, breast feeding can become a safer option for infant feeding. ART reduces the HIV viral load in the mother's blood and thereby the HIV level in the breast milk. It can also be given to the baby to reduce the risk of transmission during breast feeding.

◆ Balancing the risks

Women should always be offered voluntary counselling and HIV testing during pregnancy.

Women who test HIV negative, and those who are not tested, should be advised to breast feed exclusively for 6 months and to continue breast feeding up to 2 years or beyond. They should also give the infant nutritious family foods. If the woman is at risk of acquiring HIV then it would be best to shorten the period of breast feeding.

Advice for HIV-positive mothers who are worried about breast feeding

What advice should be given to the worried mother who is HIV positive? She may be afraid that she will pass on her HIV infection to her baby. What should she do?

If, in her situation, replacement feeding is acceptable, feasible, affordable, safe and sustainable (AFASS, *see page 237*) she may decide on replacement feeding. The mother should then avoid breast feeding completely. She should be helped and supported to give replacement feeding.

Problems associated with replacement feeding

In Africa, the most important causes of infant death in the first year of life are infectious diseases such as diarrhoea and respiratory infection, which lead to malnutrition.

These diseases are often related to the following social, economic and environmental factors:

- ◆ Lack of clean and sufficient water supplies
- ◆ Poor sanitation and unhygienic disposal of waste
- ◆ Lack of nutritious food
- ◆ Lack of fuel to boil unsafe water, such as electricity, kerosene, coal and wood
- ◆ Absence of mothers who have to leave their infants in the care of others for prolonged periods of time

◆ Very large family size and poor spacing between children

◆ Low maternal education level

◆ Poor access to health care services

And can be made worse by:

◆ Very young maternal age

◆ A seriously ill mother (e.g. a mother with AIDS)

◆ Low birth weight and/or premature birth

All babies are at greater risk of disease if they are not breast fed. In conditions of poverty, where the following circumstances apply, replacement feeding can be even more dangerous:

◆ If there is uncertain or irregular supply of the formula.

◆ If the water supply is unclean and inadequate.

◆ If the sanitation service and facilities are poor.

◆ If there is a lack of fuel or disinfectant to sterilise the feeding utensils.

◆ If the mother does not fully understand how to mix the formula, and how to correctly feed the baby with the formula.

◆ If there is poor access to health care services, especially to child health clinics.

Breast feeding is a life saver for many infants at risk from the above factors. The risks from the above may be greater than the risks of MTCT if the mother is HIV positive.

Recommending replacement feeding

If AFASS conditions are met (*see below*), then a baby can be safely and adequately fed with a breast milk substitute.

AFASS CONDITIONS

Acceptable: The mother can replacement-feed without cultural or social disapproval and is supported in her decision by family and community.

Feasible: The mother (and family) has the time, knowledge and skills to prepare the replacement food correctly and to feed the baby regularly.

Affordable: The mother (and family) can obtain and pay for the ingredients of replacement feeding, as well as fuel, clean water, utensils and soap.

Sustainable: The mother (and family) can ensure that replacement feeding will be available as long as the infant needs it.

Safe: Replacement feeds can be hygienically prepared and stored, the mother or caregiver having clean hands, using clean utensils, and being able to boil water and utensils for preparing feeds.

However, it is important that the mother recognises the dangers involved in using commercial infant formula. She should also be aware that, unlike breast feeding, it will not provide her baby with some immunity from infections.

Breast milk options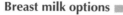

Some mothers may have the following options:

- To use an HIV-negative wet nurse who is willing to practise safe sex

- To express and boil breast milk briefly before giving it to the baby. This kills infections. The milk should be allowed to cool before feeding the baby with a cup. A cup is preferable to a bottle as it reduces the risk of infection. As a rule of thumb each feed should be 250 ml of milk for every kilogram of the baby's weight – and ideally there should be 8 feeds in the course of 24 hours

- To use pasteurised breast milk from a well-regulated milk bank

Recommending breast feeding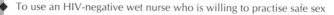

In order to reduce the risk of MTCT while breast feeding the health care worker should:

- help the mother to breast feed exclusively during the first few months

- help her stop breast feeding as rapidly as possible and only if there are safe breast milk substitutes and nutritious complementary foods available.

Help the mother to stop breast feeding by following these guidelines:

- Several weeks beforehand, show the mother how to express her milk and feed it to the baby in a cup for about 2 feeds a day.

- When you and the mother feel the time is right, she should stop breast feeding, and give all replacement feeds in a cup.

- For a while the mother can continue expressing and boiling breast milk for some feeds. This should help to avoid refusal to feed by the baby.

- The mother should continue to express milk to keep the breasts comfortable and to avoid engorgement and mastitis.

Stopping breast feeding could take place at any time up to 6 months. Ideally it should not be later than 6 months, when babies need to start complementary feeding with nutritious foods. However, breast feeding can continue a little longer if there is no other milk product available.

◆ Counselling mothers on method of infant feeding

- Counselling HIV-positive mothers on infant feeding can be difficult. It is tempting for counsellors to give advice based on their own opinions. However, it is most important to be as sensitive as possible to the mother's circumstances and wishes. Do not stress any particular method of infant feeding but help the mother to assess the risk factors carefully so she can make a proper choice.

◆ Some risk factors may be of more or less importance to the mother. Health care workers will need to use their discretion and judgement in assessing the individual situation. The mother should make the final informed choice.

Respecting and supporting the mother's feeding choice

◆ Mothers must be supported to make their own decisions about which feeding method is right for them. This should be done on the basis of full and accurate information presented in a way which she can fully understand.

◆ Mothers should not be persuaded to accept any specific feeding method.

◆ The mother's right to make her own decision must be respected. Ongoing support must be provided no matter which method she chooses. This is especially important when her decision goes against the advice that was given by the health care workers.

The health workers need to help HIV-positive mothers stop breast feeding earlier than normal and to show them how to prepare replacement feed. Ensuring that the right conditions apply for safe replacement feeding can be difficult, since these conditions depend on factors beyond the control of the health worker.

The importance of voluntary testing and counselling of pregnant women

This is outlined in more detail in Chapters 4 and 13. It should always be considered when doing HIV testing on pregnant women.

◆ Counselling and information is needed by the mother in order to make an informed and correct choice for infant-feeding methods.

◆ The mother and her partner (when appropriate) should be provided with sufficient information and counselling on the risks of MTCT and the risks of alternative methods of feeding. Only then can they make an informed choice.

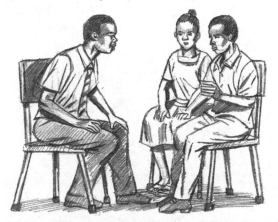

Support for HIV-positive mothers and their babies is essential.

◆ Health care workers must be careful not to have negative attitudes towards
mothers who choose a different method than that advised by the health
care worker.

◆ Accessible child health care services are strongly recommended.

◆ Sex during breast feeding

◆ Safe sexual practices are very important during pregnancy and during the breast
feeding period. Acquiring a new HIV infection during breast feeding greatly
increases the risk of transmission.

◆ If mothers and their partners wish to have sex during the breast feeding period,
they should be encouraged to use condoms to avoid new HIV infection.

For some useful websites see:

**www.who.int/child-adolescent-health/publications/pubnutrition.htm (for full list of publications
on infant feeding)**

**www.who.int/child-adolescent-health/NUTRITION/HIV_infant.htm (for access to these
documents:**

HIV and Infant Feeding: Framework for priority action

HIV and Infant Feeding: Guidelines for decision-makers

HIV and Infant Feeding: A Guide for health-care managers and supervisors

HIV and Infant Feeding Counselling: A training course

www.unicef.org/publications/index_5387.html (for helpful fact sheet on HIV and Infant feeding)

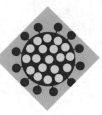

Chapter 11

AIDS AND TUBERCULOSIS

Important links between AIDS and tuberculosis (TB)

HIV testing of people with TB

Clinical considerations when managing people with HIV and TB

Managing TB patients who are co-infected with HIV

Multi drug-resistant TB (MDR)

Disseminated mycobacterial infections (MAC)

Important links between AIDS and tuberculosis (TB)

◆ HIV infection increases the risk of developing active TB

TB is the most common, serious and life-threatening opportunistic infection in people with HIV and AIDS in Africa and in other developing countries. Since the beginning of the HIV/AIDS epidemic there has been a steady increase in the number of new TB cases. The TB epidemic has shown a parallel rise. In some countries the TB epidemic has doubled and even trebled in size, and there are fears that the situation will still get worse.

Approximately 50 – 60% of people with HIV infection will develop active TB disease at some stage of their disease. This means there is a **10 times increased risk** of developing TB if a person is HIV positive.

In many parts of Africa the prevalence of HIV among people with active TB is almost 50%. This means that **a patient with TB is also very likely to have HIV infection**. Patients with HIV and TB are referred to as being **dual-** or **co-infected**.

> **The AIDS epidemic causes a parallel rise in the TB epidemic.**
> **Patients with TB disease are very likely to be co-infected with HIV as well.**

Reactivation of old TB infection or newly acquired TB infection

Immune-deficiency increases the risk of developing active TB disease due to the following:

◆ The lowered immunity in the body allows **reactivation of dormant or latent TB bacilli** which have been resident in the lungs for many years. They have usually been there since childhood, and are diagnosed by a positive tuberculin skin test. The re-activation and multiplication of these TB bacilli develops into active TB disease in the lung. It may also disseminate out of the lungs into the blood stream, and may infect other organs such as the lymph nodes, pleura, pericardium, meninges, bones and kidneys.

◆ The lowered immunity makes it more difficult for the body to resist **newly acquired TB infection,** and the active TB may be due to newly acquired TB.

TB is often due to *Mycobacterium tuberculosis* and occasionally *M. bovis* and *M. africanum*. Patients with severe immune-deficiency may also suffer from unusual forms of TB such as *M. avium-intracellulare* (MAI) which is discussed on *page 258*.

> **Immune-deficiency may result in reactivation of dormant TB bacilli**
> **or poor resistance to newly acquired TB bacilli.**

◆ The HIV/AIDS epidemic increases the spread of TB

The spread of TB, even among HIV-negative people, will be increased by the HIV/AIDS epidemic for the following reasons:

◆ HIV-infected people are more vulnerable to getting TB as discussed on the previous page. There are therefore more infected people to spread TB.

◆ TB infection may progress to active TB more rapidly in HIV-positive people. These people become infectious and are able to spread the TB.

◆ The diagnosis of TB in people with HIV or AIDS may sometimes be more difficult e.g. lower sputum positive TB (*see page 249*). This delays diagnosis and treatment of patients which results in them being infectious for longer.

◆ Recurrence of TB is more common and these patients may spread TB.

◆ Sexual partners may also be immune-deficient. This is because many of the sexual partners will also have HIV or AIDS, and they are more vulnerable to getting active TB.

◆ HIV and AIDS are very common in socio-economically stressed communities. These communities are very vulnerable to TB epidemics as well.

◆ HIV and TB make each other worse and more life-threatening

◆ In addition to the problem that HIV is a risk factor for developing active TB, both these conditions can make each other worse.

◆ The natural course of TB (untreated) in a person who has HIV may be worse and usually more severe than in HIV-negative patients.

◆ TB can also accelerate the progression of HIV to AIDS, or can worsen the AIDS condition itself.

◆ The TB can result in a lowering of the CD4 count and a rise in the HIV viral load.

◆ Important clinical features of dual HIV/AIDS and active TB infection

The following are some important factors which show how serious dual TB and HIV infection can be.

◆ TB may **occur earlier** in the HIV disease process than other life-threatening **opportunistic infections**. TB is not unusual at CD4 levels corresponding to 350 cells / mm³ or less.

◆ The **TB mortality** (likelihood of death) is increased. Studies show that the risk of dying from the TB is higher, and the risk of dying from AIDS is higher.

◆ There is a much higher chance of **extra-pulmonary TB** – the lymph glands, meninges, bone and spine, pleura and pericardium, kidney, liver, bone marrow, intestines, genital tracts, adrenal gland, joints etc.

◆ **Miliary TB** is more common.

◆ **Sputum-negative TB** is more common and this makes the diagnosis of TB more difficult.

◆ TB skin tests such as the **Mantoux test may be negative**, even in the presence of TB infection (adults).

◆ There is a higher chance of **treatment failure**.

◆ There is a higher chance of a **recurrence of the TB**.

◆ Adverse / unwanted **reactions to TB drugs** may be more likely. These may also be confused with HIV/AIDS-related conditions, such as symptoms of peripheral neuropathy, visual disturbances, skin reactions, diarrhoea.

◆ There is a possibility of **confusing the diagnosis** with other HIV-related lung conditions, such as PCP, viral and fungal pneumonia. This could cause a possible delay in treatment for these conditions.

◆ **Multiple drug resistance** has not yet been shown to increase with HIV infection. However it is still a concern.

◆ **Unusual forms of TB** such as MAI *(Mycobaterium avium-intracellulare)* are more common, especially in the advanced AIDS stage.

◆ **Drug interactions** between some TB drugs, such as rifampicin, and some HIV-related drugs, such as some Protease inhibitors are possible *(see pages 247 – 251)*.

Many of the above issues are very important considerations in the management of people with HIV/AIDS, and in managing dually infected patients (see page 247 – 251).

AIDS AND TUBERCULOSIS

Many doctors who have experience and expert knowledge in the treatment of HIV, AIDS and TB believe that every person with active TB infection should be *offered* an HIV test. There are many good reasons why it is important to know if a patient with TB has HIV infection.

Some benefits of TB patients knowing their HIV status include:

◆ The mortality from TB is higher and the patient may need to be seen more regularly.

◆ The possibility of recurrent TB is more likely. This means that more careful follow-up and counselling is necessary.

◆ The sexual partners may be HIV positive and may be vulnerable to TB. Patients may need counselling for this, and help in telling their partners / families about HIV/TB.

◆ There are conditions that are common in HIV patients which should be checked at each follow-up visit. Some conditions may be confused or missed in patients with TB, e.g. lymphadenopathy, other chronic lung conditions, various skin conditions etc. (*see Chapter 5*).

◆ Modern treatments for HIV disease may be a possibility for the patient. These can reduce their vulnerability to getting recurrent TB by improving their health status in general.

◆ Side effects from the TB drugs may be more likely. These side effects may be confused with symptoms of HIV-related diseases, and it would be useful to know if HIV is present.

◆ Ongoing diarrhoea, that commonly occurs with people with AIDS, may affect TB drug absorption.

◆ Secondary TB prophylaxis (i.e. giving a patient prophylaxis for recurrent TB) may be needed in HIV-positive individuals.

◆ More careful follow-up care can be provided which will help to control many of the problems described above.

◆ Often the patient may benefit significantly if given proper HIV care and support.

An HIV test should be offered to all patients with TB if this is possible. Full and proper pre- and post-test counselling must be provided with the HIV testing process (see Chapter 13).

All patients with TB should be offered a HIV test.
The HIV test should be done with pre- and post-test counselling.

AIDS AND TUBERCULOSIS

Clinical considerations when managing people with HIV and TB

◆ Think 'HIV' – think 'TB'

When managing a patient with HIV or TB, you should always consider both these diseases. TB often presents earlier than other life-threatening, opportunistic infections. HIV associated TB is usually associated with CD4 counts below 350 cells / mm³.

If the patient has TB, you should always be on the lookout for signs of HIV infection

◆ You should ask if:

– an HIV test has been done in the past

– there are any sexual partners who have had HIV tests
or who are known to have HIV infection

◆ You should ask about, and look for signs and symptoms which may be suggestive or diagnostic of, immune-deficiency or HIV-related disease (*see below*).

◆ Ask about previous STIs and about the person's previous sexual history.

◆ Offer an HIV test

– provide the pre- and post-test counselling
if the patient agrees to have the test.

Signs and symptoms of immune-deficiency or HIV-related diseases / conditions

Symptoms
– mouth ulcers, thrush, difficulty swallowing (candidiasis)
– history of herpes infections such as cold sores, genital ulcers, shingles (zoster)
– previous episodes of TB
– ongoing diarrhoea, cough, weight loss
– weakness, malaise
– fevers, night sweats
– itchy skin conditions, abscesses and other septic skin lesions ('acne')
– pins and needles, weakness (peripheral neuropathy)
· – repeated and ongoing diarrhoea
– history of PCP, cryptococcal meningitis, CMV retinitis, toxoplasmosis

Signs
– weight loss (ongoing and severe)
– Kaposi's sarcoma (KS)
– generalised lymph node swelling
– recurrent herpes infection
– skin conditions e.g. seborrhoeic dermatitis, tinea (fungus), folliculitis
– acute infection or oral thrush
– scars from previous herpes zoster infection (shingles)
– hairy leukoplakia on the tongue (*see page 137*)

AIDS AND TUBERCULOSIS

> **Always be on the lookout for signs of TB in patients with HIV or AIDS.**
> **Remember that TB often presents earlier than other life-threatening,**
> **opportunistic infections in people with HIV.**

If the patient has HIV, you should always be on the lookout for signs of TB

◆ You should ask if there has been any ongoing cough, chest pain, night sweats and weight loss for no other reason.

◆ You should look for signs of TB

– weight loss, sunken cheek bones

– signs of respiratory disease, such as shortness of breath, shallow rapid breathing

– signs of chest problems such as poor respiratory movement, dullness on percussion, especially the posterior bases (effusions), bronchial breath signs (cavities and consolidation), pleural rubs (pleural inflammation), crepitations (miliary TB).

◆ Always check the sputum for acid fast bacilli (AFB) if there is a productive cough.

> **In patients with HIV/AIDS it is always essential to look out for TB.**
> **It should be diagnosed as soon as possible and treated effectively.**

◆ Possibility of unusual clinical features of TB in patients with HIV

In people with HIV/AIDS, TB often presents in the usual way. However it also may present with unusual features.

Some of these unusual features are listed below

◆ The disease may be more acute, i.e. signs appearing and progressing more rapidly than expected.

◆ Sputum-negative TB is more common than in HIV-negative people.

◆ X-ray changes may be unusual and atypical (*see page 250*).

◆ Extra-pulmonary TB is more common (lymph node, liver, spleen, bone marrow, CNS etc).

◆ Rapidly progressive TB disease may occur in advanced immune-deficiency.

◆ Unusual forms of mycobacteria infect people with immune-deficiency, e.g. MAI.

◆ Diagnosing TB

Sputum for acid fast bacilli

A sputum examination for acid fast bacilli (AFB) is the most important test for diagnosing TB. A smear-positive result indicates active TB with large numbers of TB bacilli in the lungs. The patient will then be likely to spread the TB.

Remember the following:

◆ Take at least 2 specimens for TB sputum examination. If possible at least one should be an early morning specimen.

◆ Collect sputum properly:
   – ask the patient to rinse out the mouth
   – the patient should breathe in and out deeply
   – he / she should give a good cough and spit the contents into the clearly labelled specimen container.

◆ Store the specimen container in a cold place
   – a fridge is best if transport is delayed.

◆ Send the sputum to the laboratory within 4 days in a tightly closed container.

Results of AFB test

◆ If both sputum tests are positive, then start TB treatment (see page 252).

◆ If only one sputum test is positive, then do a chest X-ray
   – if the X-ray is abnormal and suggestive of TB, then treat for TB.

◆ If only one test is positive, and there are other signs of TB (weight loss, cough, sweats etc.), then start TB treatment in the immune-deficient patient.

◆ If only one test is positive, and there are no other clinical or X-ray signs of TB:
   – do a sputum culture; repeat the sputum AFB examination after 7 – 10 days, and reassess with these results
   – try a course of a broad-spectrum antibiotic, and if symptoms still persist, then treat as for TB.

TB sputum culture

◆ TB cultures are not necessary if the sputum is definitely positive for TB (AFBs).

◆ However cultures may be needed for diagnosis of sputum-negative TB in highly suspicious cases, or for diagnosis of drug-resistant TB (drug susceptibility tests)
   – drug resistance is suggested by a poor response to treatment, or a clinically deteriorating condition in spite of treatment.

◆ TB cultures may also be helpful for diagnosing some of the unusual forms of TB, or to assist in the diagnosis of drug-resistant TB.

AIDS AND TUBERCULOSIS

> **Multi drug-resistant TB is suggested by a poor response to treatment, or a clinically deteriorating condition in spite of treatment.**

Chest X-ray

Chest X-ray in HIV/AIDS is an important investigation. This is because sputum-negative TB is more commonly found in HIV-positive patients than in HIV-negative patients.

Remember the following:

◆ TB X-ray changes may be unusual or atypical in the presence of HIV / immune-deficiency. Cavitiation may not be found, and diffuse bilateral infiltrates or lobar consolidation may be present.

◆ There may be other chronic respiratory conditions such as PCP and viral and fungal disease which may be confused with TB.

◆ A base line chest X-ray is useful in the overall management of HIV (*see Chapter 5*).

Results of chest X-ray

◆ If sputum tests are negative and X-ray signs suggest TB, then ideally:
  – repeat the sputum tests
  – do a TB culture
  – and / or treat for TB if the X-rays are indicative of TB infection

◆ However if other clinical signs are also highly suggestive of TB (e.g. weight loss, cough, sweats), then treat for TB in the immune-deficient patient.

Other tissue cultures

Remember the following:

◆ Blood cultures and TB BACTEC tests are sometimes used for diagnosis of extra-pulmonary TB or for MAI complex TB.

◆ Other cultures such as stool or urine may also be used for diagnosis of GIT or urinary TB.

◆ Tissue biopsy may be used for diagnosis of extra-pulmonary TB such as lymph node, liver, bone marrow etc.

Skin tests

◆ Mantoux / PDD skin tests are not very helpful in adults from communities where TB is common. They are not usually used in the diagnosis of TB.

Managing TB patients who are co-infected with HIV

◆ Principles of management

- ◆ Treatment is the same as for HIV-negative patients.

- ◆ First-time TB patients have a different treatment regimen than second-time / failed treatment TB patients. *This is discussed on the following page.*

- ◆ A combination of drugs are always used
  - at least 6 months therapy is given to first-time patients
  - 8 months therapy is given to second-time (recurrent) or failed treatment patients.

- ◆ Treatment can be given 5 days a week, Monday to Friday, as a daily dose.

- ◆ Compliance is essential
  - unless compliance is certain, Directly Observed Therapy (DOT) is indicated.

- ◆ A definitive diagnosis (sputum and AFB or culture positive) should always be tried before commencing treatment.

- ◆ Multi-drug resistance should always be considered if a compliant and proper treatment regimen fails.

- ◆ Try and confirm sputum negativity conversion after 3 months of treatment
  - this should definitely be confirmed by 5 months.
  - if this does not occur, consider drug resistance.

> **Patients with HIV/AIDS may present with sputum-negative TB or unusual clinical presentations. Treatment for TB may need to be started even without the usual clinical and laboratory evidence.**

◆ TB treatment regimens/protocols for adults

See the chapter Children with HIV/AIDS, page 172 for childhood treatment protocols.

Note:

- ◆ TB treatment in patients with HIV/AIDS is the same as for HIV-negative patients.

- ◆ The following TB treatment protocols are provided. These may change from time to time depending on new developments and other factors.

Newly diagnosed FIRST-TIME TB infections in adult patients

6 full months of treatment is required for first-time patients. This means 2 months intensive and 4 months maintenance.

Pre-treatment body weight	2 Months Initial Phase (treatment given 5 times a week)	4 Months Continuation / Maintenance (treatment given 5 times a week)	
	Combination tablet RHZE 120 / 60 / 300 / 200 / mg*	Combination tablet RH 150 / 100 mg	Combination tablet RH 300 / 150 mg
< 50 kg	4 tabs	3 tabs	
> 50 kg	5 tabs		2 tabs
*Ethambutol 225 mg in combination is also acceptable			
R = rifampicin; H = isoniazid (INH); Z = pyrazinamide; E = ethambutol; S = streptomycin			

Re-treatment adult patients

Patients should be regarded as 're-treatment' cases if:
- they have had one or more previous active TB disease episodes
- they have had a failed course of TB treatment
- they have only had 4 months or less treatment for a previous TB disease.

8 full months of treatment is required for re-treatment patients as follows:

Pre-treatment body weight	2 Months Initial Phase (treatment given 5 times a week)		3rd Month (5 times a week)	5 Months Continuation Phase (5 times a week)			
	RHZE 120 / 60 / 300 / 200 / mg*	Streptomycin	RHZE	RH 150 / 100 mg	E 400 mg	RH 300 / 150 mg	E 400 mg
< 50 kg	4 tabs	750 mg	4 tabs	3 tabs	2 tabs		
> 50 kg	5 tabs	1 000 mg	5 tabs			2 tabs	3 tabs

Note: Streptomycin should be reduced to 750 mg per day in those older than 45 years, and should not be given to those over 65 years.

*Ethambutol 225 mg in combination is also acceptable.

Dosage of single TB drugs

If combination tablets are not available, the following individual tablets should be substituted on a daily basis as per the initial and continuation phase on previous page.

Rx

Drug name	Under 50 kg body wt	Over 50 kg body wt
Rifampicin	450 mg daily	600 mg daily
INH	300 mg daily	300 mg daily
Pyrazinamide	1 000 mg daily	1 500 mg daily
Ethambutol	800 mg daiy	1 200 mg daily

Contact your local TB control programme for treatment protocols.

◆ Monitoring progress of treatment

After 4 – 6 weeks

Within approximately 4 – 6 weeks the weight loss should have stopped, and cough and night sweat symptoms improved.

After 3 months

After 3 months sputum samples should be negative (if they were previously found to be positive). If sputum samples remain positive, then drug resistance or non-compliance should be considered. If compliance is adequate, then tests for drug resistance should be done i.e. sputum cultures and drug susceptibility (sensitivity) testing. If TB bacilli are found to be sensitive to the drugs, then continue therapy and insist on good compliance. If drug resistance is found, see multi drug-resistant TB (MDR) *on page 257.*

After 5 months

After 5 months sputum tests should be negative. If they remain positive, repeat the cultures and drug susceptibility tests and/or consult a TB specialist or local district TB officer.

**By 3 months the TB sputum tests should be negative.
They should definitely be negative by 5 months. If sputum tests
remain positive, consider poor compliance or drug resistance.**

◆ Side effects of TB medication

It is important to be aware of the possible side effects of TB drugs. This is because some of these could be confused with symptoms and signs of HIV-related disease.

The following table is a guide to the common side effects.

Side effect	Likely responsible drug	Possible confusion with HIV-related disease
Paraesthesia – peripheral neuropathy (e.g numbness, tingling, pins and needles)	INH Sometimes pyridoxine can reverse this side effect (see below*)	Peripheral neuropathy due to HIV (usually in advanced disease)
Jaundice (hepatitis)	INH, rifampicin, PZA	Viral hepatitis, TB hepatitis
Fever and rash	INH, rifampicin	HIV, skin conditions (see page 137), fevers due to HIV infection
Renal failure	Streptomycin	HIV nephropathy
Visual disturbances	Ethambutol	CMV and toxoplasma retinitis
Hearing loss	Streptomycin	–
Bleeding tendency, shock	Rifampicin	Thrombocytopaenia due to HIV

Note:
*With patients who are diabetics, epileptics, pregnant, alcohol abusers or have symptoms of peripheral neuropathy, 50 mg pyridoxine should be added to any drug regimen which includes INH.

In all of the above drug-related side effects, the drug should be temporarily or permanently stopped.

◆ ART and TB

The following needs to be considered:

 There may be shared TB and ARV drug toxicities (peripheral neuropathy, hepatitis, rash, gastro-intestinal symptoms).

◆ Commencing TB treatment may paradoxically worsen the TB disease initially (increased TB infiltrates, increased lymph adenopathy etc.). This is more common in patients who commence ART. The phenomenon is in part due to an **'immune reconstitution'**. For this reason, a delay in commencing ART in TB patients is recommended as follows:

- If the patient is already on ART, the regimen should be changed, if possible, to be compatible with rifampicin.

- If the patient's CD4 count is > 200, commence ART after completing tuberculosis therapy (providing the patient fulfils the criteria above).

- If the CD4 count is < 200, delay ART until after the intensive phase of tuberculosis therapy (2 months). This is unless the patient has other serious HIV-related illness or has a very low CD4 count – in which case ART should be introduced only once the patient is stabilised on tuberculosis therapy.

ARV interactions with rifampicin

NRTIs	No interactions
Efavirenz	Mild reduction in efavirenz levels – some experts increase the dose to 800 mg
Nevirapine	Moderate reduction in nevirapine levels – limited experience
Ritonavir (full dose)	No significant interaction
Ritonavir + saquinavir (both 400 mg 2 x daily)	No significant interaction
All other PIs	Marked reduction in PI levels – avoid

◆ **Primary prophylaxis (prevention) of TB in patients with HIV/AIDS**

A 9 month course of INH for HIV/AIDS patients has been shown to reduce the incidence of TB in these patients.

INH prophylaxis works mainly by preventing re-activation by latent or dormant TB bacilli in the lungs. For this reason it is given for 9 months only. In low TB prevalent areas, such as Europe and America, prophylaxis is usually only offered to Mantoux skin test positive patients. However this test is unreliable, and is not very helpful in countries where TB is common.

A combination of rifampicin and pyrazinamide (PZA) given for 2 months can also be used as an alternative to INH prophylaxis.

Important points about INH prophylaxis

INH prophylaxis may reduce the chance of developing active TB but its success is not certain.

It should only be considered in very compliant and reliable patients. It should not be offered to patients who may not adhere fully to the prophylaxis therapy.

It should never be given to a patient with any signs which may suggest an active TB infection. This is because it is important to avoid giving anyone with active TB only one drug (this will encourage resistance to INH).

Indiscriminate (careless) use of INH prophylaxis will promote TB drug resistance.

INH prophylaxis should not be used for routine use. It should only be offered to selective patients (*see below*).

Only certain patients should be offered INH prophylaxis

Some clinicians give the prophylaxis early in the stage of disease. Some prefer to wait:

– until the CD4 cell count is less than about 400 cells / mm^3

– or until there is clear clinical evidence of immune-deficiency

There should be no clinical signs of TB such as unexplained weight loss, chronic cough, night sweats or any other respiratory signs or symptoms. Ideally a chest X-ray should be normal to exclude the possibility of active TB.

There must be a strong chance that the patient is fully compliant with the therapy. The patient should be reliable to follow-up and be able to get on-going supplies of medication easily.

If the above criteria are met, consider offering the following for primary prophylaxis:

Rx

Dosage and duration of INH prophylaxis:

◆ INH 300 mg daily Monday to Friday

◆ Pyridoxine 25 – 50 mg daily

◆ Give treatment for 6 – 12 months (*see also page 110*)

Note: PZA (1 000 – 1 500 mg) and rifampicin (450 – 600 mg) combination daily for 2 months can also be used for prophylaxis

INH prophylaxis should only be used in selected patients who are likely to adhere to therapy. It is important that they DO NOT have any signs or symptoms of active TB (weight loss, cough, chest pain, abnormal chest X-ray).

Multi drug-resistant TB (MDR)

Drug resistance is fortunately uncommon, but it is becoming more common. It is usually due to inadequate treatment for TB or due to poor compliance by the patient. Every attempt must be made to minimise the occurrence of MDR and to effectively isolate and treat patients with MDR.

MDR is present if:

◆ The patient does not respond to treatment with a drug regimen containing INH and rifampicin.

◆ There is clinical and laboratory evidence of resistance to these drugs.

MDR is a very serious situation for the following reasons:

◆ The patient is at much higher risk for progressive life-threatening TB.

◆ The cost of treating MDR is very expensive.

◆ It could spread to others including health care personnel with severe results.

> **Inadequate or poor compliance to TB treatment is the most common cause of MDR. All cases of MDR should be referred to a TB specialist centre for correct management.**

Treatment of MDR

Treatment of MDR should continue for at least 12 months after a sputum-negative conversion. This means that the full treatment should last from 18 – 24 months. Drug susceptibility testing should guide the choice of drugs.

The following 'second-line' TB drugs can be considered for MDR:

- ethionamide 250 mg 8 – 12 hourly
- cycloserine 250 mg 8 – 12 hourly
- capreomycin 1 g daily IMI
- kanamycin 1 g daily IMI
- PAS (para aminosalicylic acid) 4 –12 g daily
- ofloxacin 400 mg 12 hourly
- ciprofloxacin 750 mg 12 hourly

> **Refer MDR patients to a TB specialist centre for investigation and therapy.**

Disseminated mycobacterial infections (MAC)

Mycobacteria avium / intracellulare complex (MAC) rarely cause disease unless the patient is severely immune-deficient. They are therefore usually found in patients with advanced stages of AIDS. These infections are often acquired via the gastro-intestinal tract as most of these organisms are environmental contaminants of soil, water, dust and aerosols.

◆ Experience with MAC is more common in countries where the usual forms of TB are uncommon.

◆ It is also not always certain whether an infection with MAC actually is causing organ damage and disease.

◆ MAC organisms are frequently found in patients without causing ill health.

◆ It is not clear whether MAC disease is due to activation of existing infection or due to newly acquired organisms.

◆ In countries with major AIDS epidemics, the incidence of MAC disease may increase significantly.

MAC disease

◆ Typically the patient is very immune-deficient with a CD4 cell count less than 50 – 100 cells / mm³.

◆ It is often associated with chronic symptoms of malaise, weakness, high fever, night sweats and weight loss.

◆ Dissemination to the lymph glands, liver, spleen and gastro-intestinal tract occur.

◆ Symptoms usually relate to which organ system is infected
e.g. lymphadenopathy, hepatosplenomegaly, diarrhoea and abdominal pain / cramps etc.

Diagnosis of MAC

◆ MAC is best diagnosed by isolation from blood (BACTEC test).

◆ Isolation from cultures of bone marrow, liver or lymph nodes may be possible.

◆ Isolation from stool and sputum may be unreliable as MAC is commonly found in these fluids in asymptomatic individuals.

◆ A high alkaline phosphatase level is often suggestive of MAC if other symptoms are also present.

Treatment

Rx

Refer to a specialised TB or HIV treatment centre / hospital.

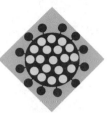

Chapter 12

SEXUALLY TRANSMITTED INFECTIONS

HIV and STIs

A practical approach to syndromic care

Some important considerations in people with HIV/AIDS and STIs

Some useful information on syphilis tests

Genital warts

Improving the quality of STI care

HIV and STIs

There is a very close relationship and association between common sexually transmitted infections (STIs) and HIV/AIDS. The care and prevention of STIs is now one of the most important and effective strategies for the control of HIV/AIDS. Numerous research studies have shown that effective community care for STIs can effectively reduce the incidence of HIV in the community. Keeping people free of STIs will also help reduce their vulnerability to getting HIV.

This chapter will briefly explore some of the important features of HIV and STIs. It will also outline the syndromic approach to managing STIs in general.

◆ STIs enhance the transmission (and spread) of HIV

There are many reasons why STIs and HIV are so closely linked. Some of these are outlined below.

STIs cause inflammation

◆ HIV is naturally attracted to the **immune cells of the body**. Many of these cells, such as CD4 lymphocytes, macrophage cells and dendritic cells, have specific receptors on their surfaces. HIV is able to attach to these surfaces and to gain entry into the cells. This is thought to be an important mechanism whereby HIV is able to infect cells and to gain entry into the body.

◆ STIs commonly cause **genital inflammation**, with a migration of many millions of inflammatory cells to the site of infection. This means that there are many immune cells with CD4 receptors in and around the genital tract. HIV can find these receptor cells much more easily in the presence of an STI.

◆ STIs (especially **genital ulcers/sores**) make it 5 to 10 times easier for HIV to enter the body through the above process.

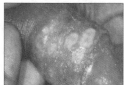

Genital ulcer

STIs cause damage to the surface and natural barriers in the genital tract

◆ STIs also disrupt the natural surfaces and linings of the genital tract. This is also thought to increase the likelihood of HIV successfully entering and leaving the body during sexual contact.

HIV is spread in the genital discharges

HIV is found in high concentration in genital discharges and secretions. Therefore if a person has HIV infection and an STI, then he / she will shed many HIV viruses in the discharge and infect others more easily. It has been shown that it is possible to reduce the amount of HIV in the discharge if the STI is effectively treated.

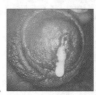
Genital discharge

> **Treating and preventing STIs will help to prevent the transmission of HIV into the body and the spread of HIV to others.**

◆ People who get STIs are also at risk for getting HIV

People who get STIs are usually having unprotected sex with different partners, or their sexual partner is having unprotected sex with other sexual partners. These are the same sexual practices that increase HIV infection and its spread.

There is a much higher prevalence and incidence of HIV among patients with STIs. Also people with HIV have higher rates of STI infections.

◆ People who have HIV also increase the spread of STIs

Immune-deficiency may delay the healing and cure of STIs

 People with HIV develop immune-deficiency.

◆ This immune-deficiency may serve to delay the healing of an STI (especially chancroid, herpes and possibly syphilis).

HIV may allow the STI to be more severe or complicated

◆ In the presence of HIV infection there is more likelihood of the STI being more severe.

 This causes larger lesions and more discharge. It also causes complications with recurrences (especially herpes infection).

HIV may result in higher chances of treatment failure

◆ In the presence of HIV infection, there is a higher chance of drug treatment failures.

 This is found especially in diseases such as chancroid and herpes.

The above individuals will be infectious for longer and will be able to spread the STI more easily.

> **Patients with HIV infection who get STIs may need more careful follow-up to ensure that the STI gets properly cured.**

◆ In the presence of an STI, always look for signs of HIV infection

Health care workers should always be on the look-out for HIV infection in patients with STIs.

If a patient has an STI it is important to consider whether he / she has HIV infection. Ideally an HIV test should always be offered to patients with STI. This however may not be possible, or the patient may not want to have an HIV test.

Looking for signs of HIV-related disease may also give clues to HIV infection.

In patients with STI always examine for:

◆ Generalised lymphadenopathy

◆ Oral thrush (and vulvo-vaginal thrush in women)

◆ Current or past Herpes zoster infection

◆ Current or past herpes infections of the skin, lips or genitals

◆ Hairy cell leukoplakia on the tongue

◆ Seborrhoeic dermatitis, skin sepsis, folliculitis

◆ Kaposi's sarcoma

◆ Recent or current opportunistic infections suggestive of HIV infection, such as TB or other recurrent or unusual respiratory infections, recurrent diarrhoea, weight loss, meningitis

◆ Recurrent illness and unwellness

> **If a patient has an STI, it is important to consider whether he / she has HIV infection.**

A practical approach to syndromic care

◆ The new 'syndromic approach' to STI management

STIs are due to many different infectious diseases, for example gonorrhoea is due to infection by the *gonococcus* bacteria, syphilis by *Treponema pallidum*, urethritis by *chlamydia*, chancroid by *Haemophilus ducreyi* etc.

There are many different organisms and diseases.

- ◆ They generally present with only a few main symptoms / signs or syndromes i.e. they either present with:
    - a discharge from the genital tract or a sore / ulcer on the genitals
- ◆ There are often other symptoms such as:
    - lower abdominal pain (usually below and / or on the side of the umbilicus)
    - burning on micturition
    - swelling of lymph glands etc.

> **The discharge or a vaginal or urethro-genital sore / ulcer is the main presenting or defining syndrome.**

◆ The old approach to STI treatment

In the past, the emphasis was on trying to make a **specific diagnosis and treating the specific disease**, e.g. if a male patient presented with a sore/ulcer or a discharge, we would try and work out which infecting organism it was caused by and treat this specifically. This would mean doing urethral swabs and other laboratory tests, and treating very specifically with a specific antibiotic.

The problems with this approach

- ◆ The clinical signs are often confusing.
- ◆ It is very difficult to clinically tell the difference between the different infections
- ◆ The laboratory tests take time and cost money.
- ◆ The patient may often not return for the follow-up.
- ◆ To complicate the matter more, the cause of the STI was often due to mixed infections of more than one different organism. The person often has one or more different infections at the same time, e.g. the sores may be due to mixed infections caused by chancroid and syphilis together.

> **STIs are often due to mixed infections, and it can be very difficult to make a specific diagnosis by clinical examination alone. Laboratory tests are costly and time consuming. Patients often do not return to get their laboratory results.**

◆ Current treatment approach to STIs

To simplify the matter we now treat the condition according to how it presents, and not according to the specific diagnosis. The process is quick and easy, and treatment is usually successful. If the presentation is for a sore / ulcer, then we give a treatment protocol appropriate to cover all the common causes of sores / ulcers and of discharge. This means that laboratory tests are not usually needed.

If the syndromic treatment fails, then the patient needs to be referred for special investigations to determine the infecting organism, and to treat with specific alternative therapies.

> **Syndromic treatment means treating the major presenting or defining symptom, such as a discharge or a sore / ulcer, with a protocol of care to cover the common causes. This is done instead of trying to make a specific diagnosis and treating the specific cause alone. The process is quick and easy and treatment is usually successful.**

Advantages and disadvantages of the syndromic approach

Advantages:

- Treatment is quick, often using a single or stat dose of drugs. This promotes improved compliance.
- The treatment regimen is designed to cover all the common causes of the syndrome.
- Expensive laboratory tests are unnecessary.
- Treatment is simple, straightforward and easily given by most primary care providers.
- Treatment successes are more common.

Disadvantages:

- Sometimes the patient gets more medication than may be necessary. This increases the cost of care. However this is often offset by the savings of not doing laboratory tests.
- Sometimes a mild vaginal discharge may be normal in a woman
  - it may not be an STI
  - some symptoms, e.g. burning on micturition may be due to a cystitis, and may not strictly be an 'STI'.
- The lack of a specific diagnosis can make contact tracing problematic, e.g. many women have a mild, non-offensive discharge which is normal. This could be interpreted as an abnormal discharge, and treatment given to the male partner unnecessarily.

On the following pages are the suggested and currently recommended treatment protocols for the different STI syndromes. Please note that treatments may differ in some areas or in some health services, and treatments may change over time.

SEXUALLY TRANSMITTED INFECTIONS

◆ Syndromic treatment of STIs

Genital (urethral) discharge
with or without swelling and painful testes

The following treatment protocol is for an abnormal, white, yellow or greenish urethral discharge.

– In males this will be from the urethra of the penis.
– In females it will be from the cervix or the urethra
 (but may appear to be coming from the vagina).

The common causes of these discharges are due to gonococci (gonorrhoea) and chlamydia (non-gonococcal urethritis), and mixed infections are common.

Treatment

Rx

Syndrome 1 – DISCHARGE FROM THE PENIS OR FROM FEMALE URETHRA / CERVIX

Ciprofloxacin 500 mg stat AND doxycycline 100 mg 12 hourly for 7 days

Alternative medication

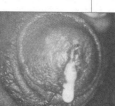

Penile discharge

◆ The following medications can be substituted if:
– the patient is sensitive to the medications above
– the patient is pregnant (ciprofloxacin and tetracycline, such as doxycycline, should not be used in pregnant women)
◆ For ciprofloxacin substitute:
– co-trimoxazole 10 tablets daily for 3 days
– kanamycin or spectinomycin 2 g IMI stat
– ceftriaxone 250 mg IMI stat
– cefixime 400 mg stat

◆ For doxycycline substitute:
– erythromycin 500 mg 6 hourly for 7 days
– tetracycline 500 mg 6 hourly for 7 days
 (not in pregnancy)
– azythromycin 1 g stat after meals

Note:

In women a discharge needs to be treated with metronidazole as well
(see Syndrome 2 on the following page).

Treatment

R̲x̲

> ## Syndrome 2 – DISCHARGE FROM THE VAGINA (i.e. not specifically from the urethra) with or without symptoms of pelvic inflammatory disease (PID)
>
> **Symptoms of PID may include:**
>
> - discharge with lower abdominal pain
> - burning on micturition
> - fever
> - often tenderness in the iliac fossae or of the cervix and adnexae on vaginal examination
>
> **Ciprofloxacin 500 mg stat AND doxycycline 100 mg 12 hourly for 7 days AND metronidazole 400 mg orally 12 hourly for 7 days. The 7 day treatment is preferable, but if patient adherence is unreliable, give 2 g stat with lots of water.**
>
> **Alternative medication**
>
> Alternative medication can be substituted (as on *page 266*) if:
>
> - there are drug allergies
>   the patient is pregnant (ciprofloxacin and tetracycline, such as doxycycline, should not be used in pregnant women)

Genital sores / ulcers

Most genital ulcers / sores are due to syphilis and chancroid. In some areas lymphogranuloma inguinale (LGV) and granuloma venereum (GV) are also common.

Herpes simplex (genital herpes) is now very common, especially in patients with HIV infection. This is discussed *on the following page.*

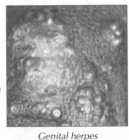

Treatment

Genital herpes

R̲x̲

> ## Syndrome 3 – GENITAL ULCER/SORE (excluding herpes infection)
>
> **Benzathine penicillin 2,4 MU IMI stat AND erythromycin 500 mg orally 8 hourly for 5 days**
>
> **Alternative medication**
>
> If allergic to penicillin, then give the erythromycin for 14 days or substitute the above with doxycycline 100 mg 12 hourly for 14 days.

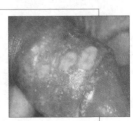

Genital ulcer

Treatment

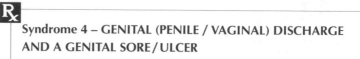

Syndrome 4 – GENITAL (PENILE / VAGINAL) DISCHARGE AND A GENITAL SORE / ULCER

Benzathine penicillin 2,4 MU IMI stat

 – AND erythromycin 500 mg orally 8 hourly
  for 5 days
 – AND ciprofloxacin 500 mg stat

Genital herpes

Genital herpes is usually a recurrent infection. It often recurs at times of physical stress, illness or around the menstrual period. The condition usually presents with small blister-like sores, which may join up to form larger sores.

Sometimes the herpes can get secondarily infected with other bacteria, and be confused with some of the genital

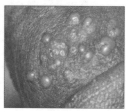
Genital herpes

ulcer diseases above. Genital herpes is usually painful, is self-limiting and settles after about 10 – 14 days.

Herpes and HIV infection

◆ In patients with HIV, herpes commonly recurs more frequently, and usually remains active and painful for longer periods.

◆ It is generally more severe than in non-HIV-positive people.

◆ It is also common to find the ulcers spreading to the perineum area and the peri-anal area.

◆ Peri-anal and genital herpes sores may join up to form large, superficial sores which do not look like the typical herpes blisters.

◆ Herpes, in the presence of HIV, can be a very difficult condition to manage. It may need a longer course of treatment.

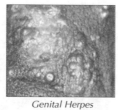

Genital Herpes   *Large superficial herpetic ulcers*

Herpes infection is very common in people with immune-deficiency.

SEXUALLY TRANSMITTED INFECTIONS

Treatment

Rx

Mild cases often do not need specific treatment and will disappear after about 10 – 14 days.

In more **severe cases,** or if there is **frequent recurrence** (especially in the presence of advanced HIV), give the following:

Valaciclovir 500 mg 2 x daily (12 hourly) for 5 days

> **or**

Acyclovir 200 mg 5 times a day for 5 days

> **or**

Famciclovir 250 mg 3 x daily (8 hourly) for 5 days

If there is frequent recurrence, give the above therapy as soon as early symptoms appear.

Suppressive therapy

If there is frequent recurrence, and the infection is severe, suppressive therapy can be offered as follows:

- – valaciclovir 500 mg daily
- – **or** acyclovir 200 mg 6 – 12 hourly

Refer any patient who gets repeated STIs or who does not respond to syndromic treatment to a urologist or specialist STI centre.

◆ Failure of syndromic treatment

If syndromic treatment fails, consider the following:

◆ The medication may not have been taken properly and completely.

◆ The sexual partner may not have been treated, and the patient is being re-infected.

◆ The STI may be resistant to the medications being offered.

◆ The patient may have HIV with immune-deficiency, and may need prolonged or more aggressive therapy.

◆ Sometimes, herpes infection, especially in the presence of HIV, may appear unusual or be secondarily infected. This can result in unusual features. Herpes will not respond to the usual syndromic protocols.

◆ The STI may be of an unusual cause, consider referring to a urologist / gynaecologist or specialist STI treatment centre for special investigation.

Some important considerations in people with HIV/AIDS and STIs

If the patient has HIV/AIDS, treat STIs as indicated on pages 266 – 269. The following points must be remembered:

- Chancroid (a genital ulcer / sore) may need treatment with erythromycin for longer periods than is recommended in Syndrome 3 (*see page 267*).

- Primary syphilis may need 3 weekly injections with benzathine penicillin, and more than just one single dose as recommended in Syndrome 3 (*see page 267*).

- Secondary and tertiary syphilis may be more common in people with HIV, and may need to be considered if symptoms are present.

- Serological tests for syphilis may be misleading and unreliable (*see also page 272*).

- The non-specific treponemal tests (RPR / VDRL) can sometimes be negative in the presence of a co-infection with HIV and syphilis
    - they also may not revert to negative after treatment.
    - if the non-specific tests do not revert to negative, then there should be a lowering of the titre.
    - if the titre is not lowered and the test has not reverted to negative, then re-treatment should be considered.

- Specific treponemal tests (TPHA / FTA-ABS) may become negative in treated patients with advanced HIV disease.

- Herpes infections may be more severe, recur more frequently, extend to the perineum or peri-anal area and appear as large sores. These infections need aggressive treatment and may need suppressive therapy (*see page 138*).

- Warts are more common in patients with HIV. Human papilloma virus, the common cause of warts, is also more common in patients with HIV
    - PAP smears for early cervical cancer detection in women should be part of the yearly routine tests.

Some useful information on syphilis tests

Serological tests for syphilis may be needed to help make a diagnosis of syphilis.

This is especially important for:

- Genital sores which may not readily heal with therapy;
- Signs of secondary syphilis (lymphadenopathy, skin rashes, condylomata, snail track ulcers on the mucous membranes etc.);
- Possible tertiary syphilis, especially in neurological diseases.

The following is a brief guide to the syphilis tests.

◆ Non-specific treponemal tests

These tests (such as RPR or VDRL) look for antibodies to the substances similar to those found on *Treponema* (the bacteria which causes syphilis). They usually become positive approximately 6 weeks after infection. In very early infection the test may therefore be negative. Non-specific tests are almost always positive in untreated primary, latent and secondary syphilis. In tertiary syphilis there may be a false negative result.

The titre

- The RPR and VDRL are also quantitative tests. The 'titre' can measure the level of antibody in the serum.
- A higher titre means there is more antibody, and indicates more likelihood of active infection.
- A dropping titre or a low titre usually indicates successful treatment.
- Titres are best evaluated by comparing them to previous values. A single titre value is often less helpful.
- After successful treatment of primary syphilis the titre should fall, and later become negative.
- In the later stages of syphilis the titre may sometimes not revert to negative. In successful treatments the titre will usually either fall or remain the same.
- Patients with HIV, especially if they are immuno-suppressed, may have active disease with very low titres or even negative reactions. This is because they are not producing antibodies as normal.

◆ Specific treponemal tests

These tests (such as the FTA-ABS and TPHA) are antibody tests to specific treponemal antigen.

- – The FTA become positive approximately 3 weeks after the initial infection.
- – The TPHA usually becomes positive 8 weeks after infection.

A positive result is recorded when titres of 1:80 or more are detected. A negative test corresponds to titres of 1:40 or less.

These specific tests usually remain weakly positive for life even after successful treatment of a syphilitic infection. They are of no value in monitoring responses to therapy.

The following table is a guide to interpretation:

RPR	TPHA	FTA – ABS	INTERPRETATION OF SERUM TESTS FOR SYPHILIS
NEG	NEG	NEG	No evidence of active treponemal infection.
NEG	NEG	POS	Early primary syphilis or long-standing (probably treated) infection.
NEG	POS	NEG	Suggests treating syphilis or false positive TPHA.
NEG	POS	POS	Suggests early treated syphilis or late untreated infection.
POS	NEG	NEG	Probable false positve.
POS	NEG	POS	Strong suggestion of primary syphilis.
POS	POS	NEG	Strong suggestion of primary syphilis.
POS	POS	POS	Confirms active or latent syphilis.

False positive results may occur in patients with other diseases or infections, e.g. malaria, abnormal globulins or positive ANF.

Patients co-infected with *T. pallidum* and HIV may demostrate both enhanced and reduced RPR reactions. Specific serology may become negative with advanced HIV disease.

(Reference: Table taken from the Laboratory Advice Form of The South African Institute for Medical Research)

Genital warts

- ◆ Genital warts are very common in people with HIV who have immune-deficiency. There are high infection rates with human papilloma virus which is also a cause of cervical cancer in women.

- ◆ Warts should be treated in the usual manner via cautery or cryotherapy with nitrous oxide.

- ◆ If the warts are few in number, podophyllin can be used.

- ◆ Podophyllin should be applied on a weekly basis until the warts disappear.

- ◆ Podophyllin should not be given to pregnant women.

- ◆ ART may also lead to the disappearance of warts.

Improving the quality of STI care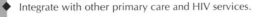

Make services accessible and user-friendly

◆ Integrate with other primary care and HIV services.

◆ Try and provide clinic services at convenient times especially in the evenings and at weekends.

◆ Syndromic care should reduce the waiting times and should speed up the care of patients.

Avoid stigma, blame and negative attitudes towards patients

◆ Treat patients with respect and dignity.

◆ Set aside one's own moral attitudes and judgements. Approach patients with a neutral attitude.

◆ Many patients are victims of circumstances, and do not choose or desire to get STIs. Do not approach them as people who have done wrong!

Advise and counsel

◆ Try to find time to counsel patients about the cause of the STIs and the need for compliance with treatment.

◆ Partners should be referred for treatment.

◆ STI patients should practise safe sex – condoms should be used until the infection is fully healed.

◆ Provide condoms at the STI clinics.

◆ If treatment does not cure the condition, the patient must be advised to return.

◆ In busy clinics it may be necessary to employ an NGO or volunteers to assist with counselling.

When to refer

◆ If the syndromic treatment fails, then the STI may need to be specifically investigated (serological tests, swabs etc).

◆ The patient may need to be referred to a more highly trained or skilled STI sexual health practitioner or reference clinic.

Remember the important C's

◆ Compliance and completeness of treatment is essential.

◆ Counsel the patient about sexual practices, partner disclosure and partner treatment etc.

◆ Condoms must be used until the STI has healed, and for the prevention of future STIs.

◆ Contacts must also be treated and counselled.

SEXUALLY TRANSMITTED INFECTIONS

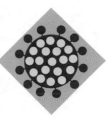

Chapter 13

COUNSELLING

The importance of counselling

Counselling and the health care worker

Counselling skills

Some common counselling needs of people
with HIV/AIDS

Referrals

The importance of counselling

HIV infection and AIDS lead to ill health and often to emotional, psychological and social problems. These problems can also cause severe difficulties with relationships. HIV/AIDS usually affects people between the ages of 15 and 50, as well as newborn babies and young children. AIDS is very much a disease of families. It also raises many difficult issues for families and even communities.

The infected people and their partners, and members of their family or close friends often need support during this difficult time.

Caring for people with HIV/AIDS calls for medical and psycho-social support.

Some of the more common psychological and social problems affecting people with HIV/AIDS include:

◆ Having an HIV test and coping with the result of the test (*see Chapter 4*)

◆ Coping with feelings of fear, guilt, anger, depression, shame and sometimes blame

◆ Adjusting to safer sexual practices

◆ Adjusting to the fact of having acquired a serious, life-threatening disease

◆ Making decisions about using costly ART

◆ Coping with the many uncertainties about AIDS

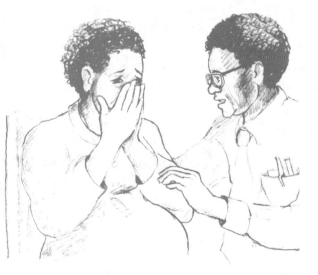

- It is often uncertain when a person became infected, or from whom.
- It is uncertain when, or if, he/she will develop symptoms of disease and what diseases these might be.
- Once he/she has the disease, it is uncertain how he/she will respond to the treatment.
- Finally, it is often uncertain for how long he/she may continue to live a normal life.
- There are many other potential uncertainties.

Problems affecting people with HIV/AIDS also include the following:

◆ Denial of being HIV-infected or of the severity of the situation

◆ Problems with relationships and family issues

◆ Making decisions on ART and adherence to ART

◆ Making decisions about pregnancies and possible termination of pregnancies

◆ Coping with an HIV-infected newborn

◆ Coping with illness and its effect, such as unemployment and sexual problems

◆ Dealing with dying, death and bereavement

◆ Coping with the loss, or future loss, of a loved one, a partner, a wife or husband, a child or a close friend in addition to their own illness

All the above issues, and many more, usually require counselling to provide the necessary psycho-social support.

◆ Why is counselling needed?

We usually solve our problems through a process of learning and experience. Sometimes we may seek help from a family member, a friend or a respected colleague. But there are times when even these people cannot help, because the problem is too big, too new, too much of a secret or too strange. When this happens, counselling can be very helpful.

Confidentiality is a major issue with HIV/AIDS. People often are too scared or too ashamed to speak to their family or friends about their condition or about their feelings and concerns.

Health care workers can provide counselling to such people, without becoming involved in their personal lives. The counsellor can offer help which is fair, objective and balanced.

Being diagnosed with HIV/AIDS, or becoming sick from the condition, often causes a crisis for the person and his / her immediate family or partner.

◆ Family and partner relationships may break down.

◆ People may think of committing suicide.

◆ Many wrong things may be done or said in this time of crisis.

A counsellor can often help to calm and stabilise people through such crises.

Finally, AIDS can cause much shame, guilt and embarrassment. Counselling can help a client (patient) to feel easier, to overcome such feelings and to face the world with confidence and dignity again.

◆ What is counselling?

The counsellor and the client together explore the issues and problems, and find new or different approaches to dealing with them. Sometimes solutions are found, but sometimes this is not possible. However, often just talking about the problem, and expressing it, will help to relieve much of the burden. Clients often only need emotional support and an opportunity to express or 'open up' their feelings and emotions.

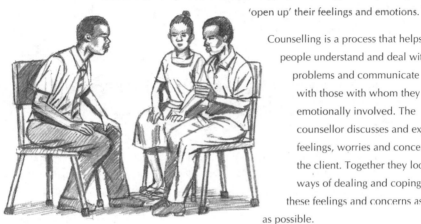

Counselling is a process that helps people understand and deal with their problems and communicate better with those with whom they are emotionally involved. The counsellor discusses and explores feelings, worries and concerns of the client. Together they look at ways of dealing and coping with these feelings and concerns as best as possible.

> **Counselling does not involve merely giving advice.**
> **It also does not mean you take over the client's problem.**
> **It means you encourage the client to find his / her own solutions to problems,**
> **and this helps him / her to become a confident and independent person.**

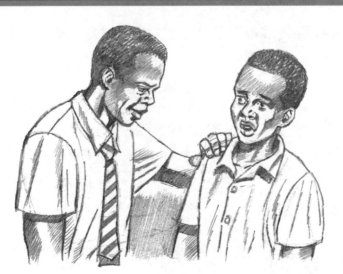

Counselling and the health care worker

Mental health care providers, such as psychologists, psychiatric nurses, social workers and psychiatrists are specifically trained to counsel people with complex problems. However, primary health care workers can become effective counsellors through training. Counselling is usually part of the normal medical consultation and should be an essential part of the care of people with HIV/AIDS.

Counselling should be confidential, professional and non-judgemental.

◆ You need to respect the confidence of your client, and in turn he/she will learn to trust and confide in you.

◆ It is a professional relationship and **not** a friendship. Friends usually get over-involved in the problems, but counsellors can maintain a controlled relationship with clients and provide a more balanced and objective approach.

◆ Accept your client for what he/she is and not what you would like him/her to be. Avoid judging your client. A client who feels judged will not feel free to 'open up' about feelings and concerns.

> **Health care workers can provide effective counselling.**
> **They must be confidential, professional and non-judgemental.**

Counselling skills

A thorough explanation of the techniques and skills for providing good counselling is not possible in this book. However, being a good listener and being able to explore the feelings, fears, worries and concerns with the client is possible for most health care workers.

Care, understanding and empathy are normal human skills.

Empathy is seeing the world through the client's eyes or from his / her point of view.

Being empathetic helps you to understand your client much better.

◆ Some tips for effective counselling

◆ **Try to find extra time** to counsel. It is very difficult to rush counselling, and you may need to set aside special time.

◆ Try to **find a private place** where you will not be interrupted.

◆ **Discuss the purpose** of the counselling, so that both of you work towards the same goal.

◆ **Avoid rushing in with advice**. It is best for the problem to be fully explored and for the client to work out possible solutions.

◆ **Listening carefully** is the most important aspect of counselling. If you listen 'actively' you will hear what the client is feeling, and what his / her main problems are. Try to spend more time listening than speaking.

◆ While listening, you should also keep **checking and communicating with the client to make sure you are receiving the correct message**. It is important to **maintain good eye contact** and to communicate back. This shows that you are understanding the feeling.

Try to find a word, or a short explanation, which best describes what he / she is saying and 'reflect this back'. Allow him / her to correct you or make the issue more clear, e.g.

Client "I don't know how I am going to tell my partner about this result."

Counsellor "It seems that you are very anxious" (the feeling) "because you do not know how your partner will react to your positive HIV test" (the situation).

Here you have acknowledged the feelings and you are putting them in context. You are also showing empathy.

◆ **Constantly check that you are hearing him / her correctly, e.g.**

Client "I am not sure what will happen to me when I get very sick".

Counsellor "So are you saying that the main problem is your fear of dying?"

◆ If you are not sure about something that he / she has said, then make this clear e.g.

Counsellor "When you said 'what will it be like when I get very sick?', did you mean what will happen to your body or to your family or.....?"

◆ Try to **analyse** and work out why the client needs help, and what the **real issues and problems are.**

◆ There is no set way to counsel. The counsellor must allow the client to **express his / her own problems** which will then form the basis for the counselling.

Tips for effective counselling continued:

◆ Ask **open-ended questions** rather than closed questions. This encourages him / her to discuss answers which you are not expecting, e.g.
Open-ended question: **Counsellor** "How is your marriage?"
(This will help him / her to talk.)
Closed question: **Counsellor** "Is your marriage good?"
(People often answer this sort of question with a simple "yes" or "no".)

◆ From time to time you should **summarise** the situation. This is a useful way of making sure that you have heard everything correctly, and it helps your client to think of the main issues.

◆ If the problem is complex, try to **break down the problem** into smaller sub-problems. Then explore each sub-problem in turn.

◆ **Not all problems are solvable**. But remember, often just talking about the problem and sharing fears, worries and concerns helps a client to cope.

◆ Remember to allow and encourage the client to **express his / her feelings**. Crying, sobbing or angry outbursts are ways people express feelings and unburden themselves.

◆ Watch how the client sits, speaks, reacts, his / her facial expressions etc. This is called '**body language**'. Body language can tell you a lot about how the client is feeling. A client who does not look you in the eye may be feeling ashamed, guilty or very anxious. A client sitting very tightly, arms folded, legs folded etc. may be feeling tense and unrelaxed.
If you notice this body language, then communicate this with him / her, e.g.
Counsellor "Are you feeling tense?" or "It seems that you are very anxious."

◆ Add to the communication programme by letting him / her know that **you are listening and in touch.**
You do this by nodding, using facial expressions, sitting relaxed but interested. Use phrases like:
"Yes, carry on";   "I see, and then?";   "I am with you";   "I hear you".

◆ **Show your support** for his / her decisions, and leave it open for the client to return for follow-up or further counselling.

◆ Sometimes it is useful to make a **short-term plan of action** for the period before the next counselling / consultation session.

Leading questions

You may also have to ask some leading questions to get the client to express his / her feelings, worries and concerns.

> **Below are some examples of leading questions:**
>
> "How are you feeling inside?"
>
> "How does that make you feel?"
>
> "Do you ever think of this by yourself?"
>
> "What kind of things do you think about?"
>
> "Who do you talk to about your condition?"
>
> "Could you share with me some of your inside feelings?"
>
> "Could you share with me your feelings or thoughts about.....?"
>
> "If your test result is positive what then?"
>
> "Now that your HIV test is positive, how does it make you feel?"
>
> "If you had to draw your feelings, what would you draw?"

Useful phrases

Also you may need to use some useful phrases to encourage him / her to talk and to show that you are listening carefully.

> **The following are examples of useful phrases:**
>
> "That's very interesting – tell me more".
>
> "I hear what you are saying – tell me more".
>
> "Can I just check with you that I am understanding the problem?"
>
> "In other words are you saying ....?"
>
> "So does this make you feel ....?"
>
> "You asked me how long I think you will live? ...do you often think of dying?" or ..."How long would you like to live?"
>
> "Are you afraid?"
>
> "Have you had enough?"

◆ Acquiring counselling skills

Most health workers need some extra training in being an effective counsellor. If possible, you should try to arrange for an experienced counsellor to provide some extra training. There are also courses that are run for this purpose.

It is also a good idea to ask your local social worker or clinical psychologist, or others experienced in counselling, to run a short workshop. In the workshop you could 'role-play' situations and practise counselling skills.

Finally, it is useful to get a supervisor with whom you can discuss your counselling problems and learn ways to deal with these. It is also useful to set up a support group for people doing AIDS counselling, to share ideas, worries, concerns and ways of dealing with difficult situations.

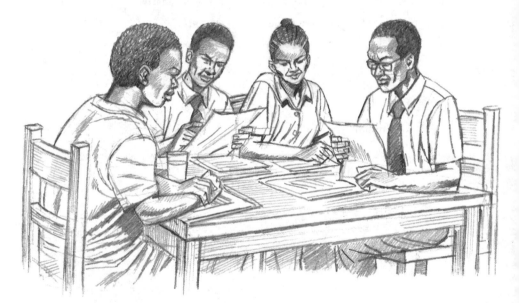

It is important for health care workers to get some extra training in counselling skills. It is also useful to have a support group where you can share ideas and concerns.

Some common counselling needs of people with HIV/AIDS

◆ Pre- and post-test counselling

The test can raise many issues and fears. Your client usually needs to discuss these before and after the test. *These are discussed in Chapter 4. Examples of interviews for pre- and post-test counselling are also given in Chapter 4 on pages 51 – 54.*

◆ Relationships

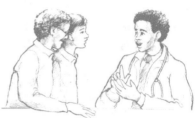

HIV/AIDS can cause many problems for people in their relationships with their loved ones, families and friends. Your client may need to talk about how and to whom he can tell that he is HIV positive. HIV-positive people often fear rejection or blame from their partners, and they may have feelings of guilt, shame, etc. Re-establishing trust may be important.

> **Counselling is often required to help deal with the feelings of rejection, guilt, shame and blame in a relationship.**

◆ Living with uncertainty

There are often many unanswered questions for people with HIV/AIDS.

Common uncertainties include:
"From whom did I get the infection?"
"When will I become ill?"
"Will I get AIDS?"
"What illnesses will I get?"
"Will there be any treatment for me?"
"Will ART be effective?"
"For how long will ART be effective?"
"For how long will I live?"
"How will people react when I tell them I am HIV positive?"

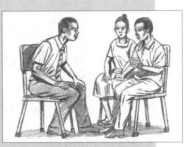

> **Uncertainty often makes people anxious and depressed.**

◆ Discrimination and rejection

People affected by HIV/AIDS are often subjected to discrimination and rejection by their friends, work colleagues, insurance schemes, and even family and partners. Support and counselling and even legal advice may be needed.

◆ HIV care options

There are now various choices available for ART. This therapy can prevent the deterioration of the disease, and can promote and maintain health. The therapy is often costly, however there are very important benefits which can prolong good life and prevent AIDS. These issues will need to be considered.

◆ Difficulties taking ARV medication and other chronic medicines

It is critical that patients on ARV medication adhere very strictly to the dosage and frequency of taking the medication. The drugs have to be taken every day on an ongoing basis.

Successful adherence to therapy is usually associated with:

- More simple drug regimens
- Daily or 12-hourly dosing frequency
- As few drugs as possible
- Understanding the need for the medication
- Support from loved ones or partners
- Fewer side effects
- As little disruption to normal routine as possible

Counselling is often required to help patients:

- Understand the need to adhere to taking the drugs regularly and without fail
- Recognise symptoms of side effects
- Comply with regular follow ups
- Cope with the frustration of needing to take medication
- Take their medication daily

◆ Pregnancy

Pregnancy raises many questions for HIV-positive people *(see Chapter 9)*. Affected people need to make important decisions.

They need to decide:

- whether to have another child or not
- whether to take ART during pregnancy to help prevent MTCT
- sometimes whether to terminate a pregnancy

There is often anxiety in pregnancy about the risk to the mother or the health of the newborn baby. It is often uncertain whether the baby is HIV positive and it may take up to 18 months to finally find this out *(see Chapter 8)*. Mothers and fathers may experience feelings of guilt and anger if their baby is HIV positive or when their baby becomes ill or dies.

People facing these and other issues need counselling and support. There are now many effective strategies to help reduce MTCT *(see Chapter 10)*.

◆ Infant feeding

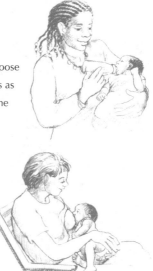

Breast feeding can transmit HIV to a baby.

A mother in Africa who has HIV is most likely to choose to breast feed. She will have major fears and worries as to whether her child will acquire HIV infection. Some mothers may choose to formula feed their babies and may be criticised for doing so by their friends, family and mother / mothers in-law. Mothers will therefore need supportive counselling and advice on how to reduce the risk of transmitting the infection to their infants.

See Chapter 10 for more on infant feeding.

◆ Sex and sexuality

Being HIV positive often means having to make major changes to one's sexual behaviour and/or the way one has sex. This, in itself, can be extremely difficult and can stress relationships with lovers and partners.

HIV infection may also mean having to come to terms with homosexuality. This may mean being open about homosexuality for the first time.
This may be a difficult and trying process.

> **HIV-positive men and women may need to adjust to different ways of relating sexually to each other.**

◆ Fear, loneliness, anger, guilt, shame and blame

Those living with HIV will experience many emotions which may be confusing and scary, such as anxiety, depression and hopelessness. Counselling can help explore many of these feelings.

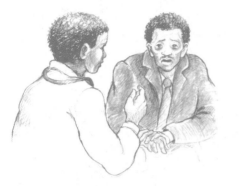

◆ Coping with illness

The counsellor needs to support the client (and often his / her loved ones as well) through the repeated illnesses and deterioration in health. You may have to help your client look at ways of living **each day**, rather than thinking too far ahead into the future.

You may have to explore ways of making the *quality* rather than the *quantity* of life better.

> **It is important to counsel clients and help them cope with loss.**

◆ Coping with losses

People with HIV suffer many losses. They lose their health, their independence and many years of life. They may also lose their lover or spouse, their job, their financial security and their usual life and lifestyle. They need to change their sexual habits. Many lose their pregnancy (through termination or abortion) and also their newborn babies.

◆ Denial

People with HIV infection often have great difficulty believing or accepting that they have a serious condition. This often results in people not returning for follow-up or continuing with unsafe sexual practices.

Counselling may be difficult if there is denial. However, it is very important in helping a client accept his/her HIV infection. Counselling will help the client develop a responsible and positive attitude.

> **Denial of one's HIV infection is a method some people use to cope with the problem.**

◆ Death, dying and bereavement

AIDS is a terminal disease and health workers will frequently be required to counsel a patient about death and dying. The partner, family and friends will also need some help.

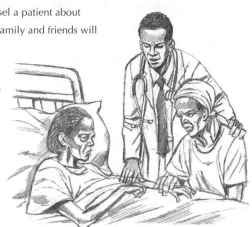

Parents lose their children and children also lose their parents. Grandparents sometimes lose their own son or daughter, and sometimes grandchildren as well.

Later, dealing with those left behind after the death, such as family members, lovers and friends, may also be necessary.

Special counselling may be needed for children who lose a parent or sibling.

Managing patients who are dying is discussed in Chapter 14.

Counselling may also be needed for children, grandparents, families, lovers and friends.

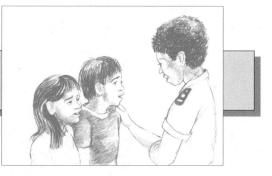

Referrals

You may find that you are not coping with a client, or the issues and problems are too complex and difficult. You may need to refer such clients to a more experienced counsellor or to someone who has more time for counselling. Try to find out who is available and willing to help counsel people with HIV/AIDS in your area and use these facilities.

The next chapter deals in more detail with the care of people who are in pain and discomfort or are dying.

Find out if your country has an AIDS Helpline and what the contact details are.

Additional notes for new developments

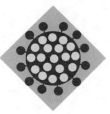

Chapter 14

THE CARE OF PEOPLE WHO ARE IN PAIN, DISCOMFORT OR ARE DYING

Pain, discomfort, anxiety and sleep problems

Some common causes of discomfort and their management

Sedation

Managing a patient who is dying

Involvement of other agencies and health care workers

Pain, discomfort, anxiety and sleep problems

Pain, discomfort, anxiety and sleep problems are common in people with conditions associated with AIDS. Health workers are also having to manage more and more patients who are dying (especially in younger age groups).

This chapter will briefly outline some useful and important ways of managing and coping with these problems.

◆ Pain and discomfort

Almost all pain can be effectively managed. It is important to attempt, as far as possible, to diagnose and treat the actual cause of the pain or the discomfort, such as nausea, vomiting, abdominal cramps, constipation headache, sleep problems etc.

If patients are in the terminal stages of HIV infection, it is important not to simply accept that all pain is due to the HIV infection alone. Try to determine if there is any new development which may respond to effective treatment.

Pain is also influenced and altered by the patient's mental and psychological state. The care of pain goes beyond drug treatment alone. It is equally important to explore the nature of the pain with the patient and his/her relatives or carers. Carefully and simply explain the cause of the pain and how you are going to relieve it. Often other worries and fears seem to make the feeling of pain even worse.

Counselling and exploring any fears, worries or concerns with the patient will often contribute to relieving pain. *Counselling is discussed in more detail in Chapter 13.*

Pain is also often worse at night and when the patient is alone. This frequently causes sleeping problems which highlight the feeling of pain and cause the patient to feel worse. Managing sleep problems and helping to ensure adequate sleep is very important in the management of pain.

> **Pain is often felt more at night and causes sleep problems. Managing pain helps to ensure sleep, which in turn helps to manage the pain.**

At night patients often lie awake and think about what is happening to them. Sometimes there is fear of not waking up again. The patient may avoid sleeping at night because of this and rather sleep in the day when people are around to wake him up. This fear, uncertainty and lack of adequate sleep can make the pain worse at night.

Other forms of comfort can help to relieve pain:

◆ Simple massage, caressing or gently rubbing parts of the body may help.

◆ Gentle music may be soothing.

◆ Traditional and home-remedies should be encouraged and used if effective.

◆ Keeping the patient company, talking and listening helps take the attention away from the pain.

◆ Treating pain

Different drugs and therapies are available for different types of pain.

Try to follow these simple rules:

◆ **Try to determine the type of pain** and the possible **cause** of the pain.

◆ **Explain the cause of the pain** and the treatment plan to relieve the pain.

◆ When using pain-relieving medication, always **first try to use oral ('by mouth') agents.** Injections and drips can cause pain themselves.

◆ Use a **'ladder' approach** to the choice of drugs. Always **start with the mildest or weakest agents first**. Slowly move up the ladder with more moderate agents and then to the more powerful and stronger agents, **depending on the patient's needs** *(see diagram on the following page).*

◆ **Treat by the clock**. Pain is suffering and therefore do not wait for the onset of pain before giving the medication. Give medication in time to prevent the return of the pain. Medication should best be given on a regular basis, such as every hour, 2 hourly, 4 hourly etc. or even by continuous infusion if necessary, rather than on a 'prn' (as required) basis. It is important to continually review the therapy. There may be 'breakthrough pain' with a need to increase dosage or frequency of the drugs, or to change to a stronger agent etc.

◆ If **movement** of a limb causes pain, it may be relieved with the aid of a **splint,** such as a plaster slab, wooden plank, rolled up newspaper etc.

> **Anti-retroviral therapy (ART) may improve the immune status and reverse various HIV–related conditions which cause pain.**

Simple rules continued:

◆ **Relieving discomfort,** such as **nausea, vomiting, constipation** etc., often helps to relieve pain. Remember also that analgesics (pain-relieving drugs) may cause constipation, especially codeine- and morphine-containing drugs. Other drugs, such as zidovudine (Retrovir), didanosine (Videx) and many others, may cause nausea, vomiting, abdominal discomfort, headache etc.

Always be on the look-out for these drug-related side effects.

Use of analgesics (pain-relieving drugs)

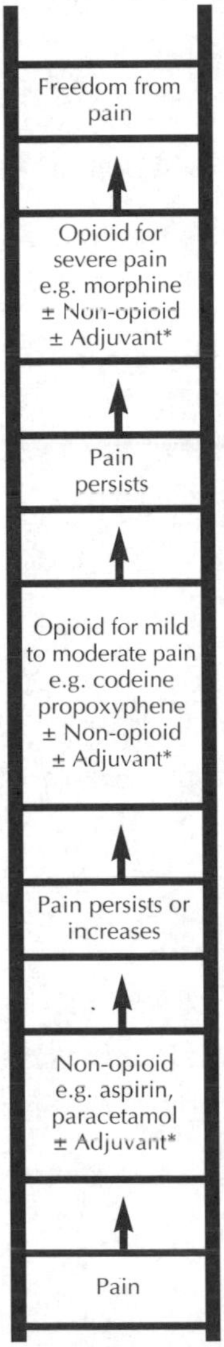

Pain-relieving drugs should be given by the following means:

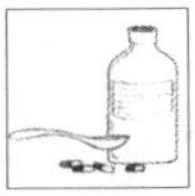

By mouth if possible.

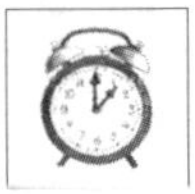

By the clock. Persistent or ongoing pain needs preventive therapy. This means that analgesics should be given regularly. You should not wait for symptoms of pain to return before giving the next dose.

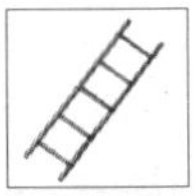

By the 'ladder'. This means that you should start with the simplest and weakest drugs and go 'up the ladder' in terms of strength.

The 'ladder' approach

Non-opioids (e.g. aspirin, paracetamol) can be thought of as 'tissue-acting analgesics' and opioids (e.g. codeine, dihydrocodeine, morphine) as 'centrally (brain)-acting analgesics'.

◆ First try simple **non-opioid** analgesics, e.g.
  – aspirin
  – paracetamol
  – ibuprofen

◆ Next try the **weaker opioids,** e.g.
  – codeine and aspirin (Codis)
  – codeine and paracetamol (Paracodol)
  – codeine by itself
  – dihydrocodeine (DF118)

  N.B. Use laxatives with these drugs

◆ Next try the **stronger opioids**, e.g.
  – dextropropoxyphene (Doloxene)
  – pentazocine (Sosenol)

The ladder diagram (left margin):

Freedom from pain

↑

Opioid for severe pain e.g. morphine ± Non-opioid ± Adjuvant*

↑

Pain persists

↑

Opioid for mild to moderate pain e.g. codeine propoxyphene ± Non-opioid ± Adjuvant*

↑

Pain persists or increases

↑

Non-opioid e.g. aspirin, paracetamol ± Adjuvant*

↑

Pain

*Note: ± Adjuvant = with or without use of other pain-relieving methods e.g. by relieving nausea, using splints, giving co-analgesics *(see page 299)* etc.

◆ Next try the **strongest opioids** e.g.

These are listed in order of analgesic strength (potency) e.g.

- tilidine (Valoron)
- dipipanone (Wellconal)
- papaveretum (Omnopon)
- morphine

N.B. Use laxatives with these drugs.

Remember laxatives must be given when using analgesics, especially the opioids. Anti-emetics may also be required.

◆ Drugs and dosage

Codeine (Phosphate)

30 mg tablet

25 mg / 15 ml syrup

Dose:

◆ Adults 15 – 60 mg, 4 – 6 hourly

◆ Children 0,5 mg/kg, 4 – 6 hourly

Pentazocine (Sosenol)

50 mg tablets and 30 mg/ml injection

Dose:

◆ 25 – 50 mg, 4 – 6 hourly orally

◆ 30 – 60 mg, 3 – 4 hourly, IMI or subcutaneously

(Maximum dosage 360 mg/24 hrs)

Not recommended for children under 12 years.

Dextropropoxyphene (Doloxene)

100 mg tablets (equivalent to 65 mg dextropropoxyphene)

Dose:

◆ Give 1 – 2 tablets (capsules) 4 hourly

(Maximum dosage 390 mg (6 capsules/24 hours)

Not recommended during pregnancy and avoid if liver or renal disease.

Dihydrocodeine (DF118)

30 mg tablets and 50 mg/ml injection. This analgesic is approximately 15% ($\frac{1}{6}$) the strength of morphine.

Dose:

◆ 30 – 60 mg tablets, every 4 – 6 hours (or more frequently if required)

◆ 50 mg IMI, 4 – 6 hourly (or more frequently if required)

◆ Children (over 4 years) 0,5 – 1 mg/kg, 4 – 6 hourly

N.B. If large doses are needed, it may be best to change to morphine.

Tilidine (Valoron) ▮▮▮▮▮▮▮▮▮▮▮▮▮▮▮▮▮▮

50 mg tablets; 50 mg/0,5 ml drops; 100 mg/2 ml injection

Dose:

◆ Tablets, drops or by injection 50 –100 mg, 4 – 6 hourly

◆ Children 1 drop for each year of age, 3 – 4 hourly (maximum 10 drops)

Side effects:

Tilidine may cause mood alteration, disorientation and hallucination.

Dipipanone (Wellconal) ▮▮▮▮▮▮▮▮▮▮▮▮▮▮▮▮▮▮

30 mg tablets

Dose:

◆ Give ½ – 3 tablets, every 4 – 6 hours

Side effects:

Dipipanone may cause confusion and/or hallucinations.

Papaveretum (Omnopon) ▮▮▮▮▮▮▮▮▮▮▮▮▮▮▮▮▮▮

10 mg/0,5 ml; 20 mg/ml (by injection only)

Dose:

◆ 10 – 20 mg IMI, 4 – 6 hourly

◆ Children 1 – 5 years 2,5 – 5 mg, 4 – 6 hourly

◆ Children 6 – 12 years 5 – 10 mg, 4 – 6 hourly

Morphine ▮▮▮▮▮▮▮▮▮▮▮▮▮▮▮▮▮▮

Morphine is available in an injectable form and in slow release tablets called MST (morphine sulphate tablet) and a morphine suspension can be used. Pain control experts prefer using a morphine suspension made up in the pharmacy (*see next page*) for oral use.

Morphine MST tablets

10 mg and 30 mg tablets.

Morphine MST is a slow releasing tablet. One 10 mg tablet is equivalent to 3,3 mg of pure morphine given 4 hourly. One 30 mg tablet is equivalent to 10 mg of morphine given 4 hourly.

Therefore you may need to give higher doses of the MST to achieve the same analgesic effect as the injection or the suspension solution *described on the next page*.

Dose:

◆ 10 – 60 mg, 4 – 12 hourly orally

N.B. Morphine MST is expensive.

Morphine suspension

A preferred oral morphine suspension can be made up in the dispensary or by a pharmacist as follows:

- Morphine sulphate powder   4 g
- Sucrose (sugar)   400 g
- Spirits of chloroform   40 ml
- Distilled water to make solution   1 000 ml

The above morphine mixture will give 20 mg/5 ml.

Further dilutions can be made up for use with children. It is best to use the suspension above.

Dose of suspension:

- 10 – 30 mg, 4 – 6 hourly
- Children: 0,1 – 0,2 mg/kg per dose, 4 – 6 hourly

Note: A 12 hourly MST dose may be a more convenient dose (see dose equivalent above). The MST is also useful to control night pain (due to its slow release) which avoids the need to wake up for a more frequent dose when using the suspension. However, MST is more expensive than the suspension.

Morphine injection

Morphine can also be given by injection subcutaneously or intramuscularly.

Dose:

- 5 – 15 mg, every 4 – 6 hours
- Children: 0,1 – 0,2 mg/kg per dose, 4 – 6 hourly

Side effects are constipation and sedation. It should not be used in pregnancy.

N.B: The correct morphine dose is that dose which relieves the pain and gives the patient the best quality of life.

> **Remember:** Opioid analgesics commonly cause constipation.
> If necessary, this should be prevented with simple laxatives.
> Also nausea and vomiting may occur, especially after starting therapy.
> Prevent constipation with control of diet or with laxatives.
> Anti-emetics are often needed when starting therapy with opioids.

> **The correct drug and the correct dose is that which relieves the pain.**
> **Too often the wrong drug is used, the dose is too little or the dose is given too seldom to effectively relieve the pain.**
> **Addiction is not a consideration in people with terminal illness.**

Co-analgesics

Some medications are very useful when used in combination with analgesics:

◆ **Non-steroidal anti-inflammatory agents (NSAIDs)**

These are mildly analgesic and inhibit prostoglandin activity. Prostoglandins promote bone and connective tissue pain, and NSAIDs are very useful for bone and joint pains. *This is discussed in more detail on page 301.*

◆ **Steroids**

Steroids are useful for reducing oedema and inflammatory reactions and therefore ease pressure on surrounding structures e.g. headache, nausea or vomiting secondary to raised intracranial pressure, bone pain, pleuritic pain, nerve and cord compression.

◆ **Muscle relaxants**

Muscle spasm due to nerve involvement may make pain worse. It may be relieved with local heat or massage. Diazepam (Valium), especially when given at night, is a useful muscle relaxant.

◆ **Central nervous system-acting drugs**

Anxiety often complicates the feeling of pain. Medication to relieve anxiety is therefore often useful e.g. diazepam (Valium), haloperidol (Serenace), amitriptyline (Tryptanol).

Phenothiazines may be combined with an opioid analgesic.

Anti-depressants can also be effective in pain associated with nerve destruction (such as pain associated with Herpes zoster). Amitriptyline is the drug of choice *(see page 301).*

Anti-convulsants, such as sodium valproate (Epilim) and carbamazepine (Tegretol), are also helpful in treating shooting nerve pains *(see page 301).*

Ten important rules/guidelines for pain control

◆ Do not assume that the pain is due to the HIV infection (think of other possible treatable causes).

◆ Try non-opioids first.

◆ Do not be afraid to use narcotic/opioids if the non-opioids do not relieve the pain.

◆ Prescribe adequate amounts of the analgesics at adequate frequencies to relieve the pain.

◆ Give the analgesic at regular intervals and avoid giving the analgesic prn (as required).

◆ Consider using co-analgesics if indicated.

◆ Use laxatives when using most of the analgesics, especially the opioids. Anti-emetics are also often needed with opioid therapy.

◆ Consider the patient's feelings and keep him/her well informed. Provide support for the family/lover/partner.

◆ Do not limit your approach to the use of drugs only.

◆ Do not be afraid to ask a colleague for advice.

CARE OF THE DYING

Some common causes of discomfort and their management

◆ Abdominal cramps and constipation

Abdominal cramps, with or without diarrhoea, may cause discomfort.

Try to exclude treatable infections, such as amoebiasis, giardiasis, salmonella and shigella.

> **Rx**
>
> ***See page 131* for the management of diarrhoea.**
>
> ◆ Antispasmodics, such as hyoscine butylbromide (Buscopan) given 8 – 12 hourly, can be used.
>
> ◆ Belladonna (tincture) is also useful.
>
> ◆ Constipation can be treated with laxatives, such as magnesium hydroxide, faecal softeners (liquid paraffin), Milpar (magnesium hydroxide combined with liquid paraffin), lactulose (Duphalac), bisacodyl (Dulcolax), senna (Senokot) and enemas (with caution).

◆ Nausea and vomiting

In HIV infection nausea and vomiting may be due to:

◆ Gastro-intestinal infection

◆ Constipation or irritation

◆ Raised intracranial pressure (cerebral infection, tumours, HIV infection)

◆ Side effects of drugs

◆ Often for unknown reasons

◆

> **Rx** ◆ Useful anti-emetic medications include prochlorperazine (Stemetil), cyclizine (Valoid), chlorpromazine and metoclopramide (Maxalon).
>
> ◆ Haloperidol (Serenace) 5 mg nightly is also useful for severe cases.
>
> ◆ Dexamethasone 4 – 8 mg IMI can also be used for very severe cases which do not respond to the above medications.

◆ Peripheral neuropathy

Peripheral neuropathy causing shooting pains, numbness, tingling, pins and needles etc. is common in people with HIV infection. Neuropathy caused by Herpes zoster (shingles) is also common.

Always try to exclude treatable disease of the central nervous system, especially syphilis, varicella zoster, CMV viral infection and other causes of meningitis or brain abscess. Some drugs, particularly isoniazid (INH), ddI (Videx), ddC (HIVID), ethambutol (and also alcohol), may cause neuropathy.

Rx

◆ Where a specific cause cannot be found or when there is a very severe shooting pain (e.g. with shingles), try carbamazapine (Tegretol) 200 mg, 8 hourly.

◆ If the pain is a burning sensation, then try amitryptiline (Tryptanol) 50 – 75 mg orally, daily.

◆ Simple analgesics do not usually help. If the pain is very severe, morphine or morphine-like agents, together with the above drugs, may be required.

◆ Headache

Headache may be due to tension, intracranial infection, intracranial tumour, cerebral oedema, side effects of drugs etc.

Rx

◆ Try to find and treat the specific cause (*see page 148*).

◆ Give analgesics.

◆ Dexamethasone 16 – 24 mg in divided doses can be used and tailed off after 2 – 3 weeks for cerebral oedema and raised intracranial pressure (discontinue after 6 days if there is no response to the therapy).

◆ Bone pain

Bone pain is more common with malignant conditions.

Rx

◆ Bone pain responds best to non-steroidal anti-inflammatory agents (NSAIDs), such as aspirin, ibuprofen (Brufen), indomethacin (Indocid), diclophenac (Voltaren), piroxicam (Feldene), naproxen (Naprosyn) etc.

◆ In very severe cases give dexamethasone 1 mg – 2 mg, 12 hourly (and increase dose if needed).

◆ Itching (pruritis)

Pruritis may be caused by dry skin or by side effects from drugs, liver or kidney disease, various skin conditions, lymphoma or the HIV itself.

R₂

Try to find the cause and treat it.
Otherwise the following is recommended.

General measures:

- Treat the dry skin (common in terminally ill patients) by advising the patient not to sit too close to a fire or heater.
- Apply wet, cool compresses to the worst affected areas.
- Ung emulsificans aqueous (UEA) can be applied to the itchy areas 6 – 8 hourly.
- Add a tablespoon of UEA to the bath water or use a bath oil, such as EABS or Johnson & Johnson baby oil. Dry the skin after the bath by patting with a soft towel.
- Oil the skin after bathing, with an emollient cream (UEA), body oils or lanolin.

Specific measures:

- Inflamed areas can be treated with a hydrocortisone/clioquinol (Vioform) preparation, such as Betnovate C or pure mild hydrocortisone creams applied 8 – 12 hourly.
- Hydrocortisone in menthol (1:3) is also useful.
- Antihistamines can be tried in severe cases but are often of little help.
- A short course of oral steroids may also relieve severe symptoms.

Note: Usually the most effective way to manage pruritis is by preventing and managing the dry skin.

Sedation

Sedation is often needed late in the course of HIV disease for sleep problems, discomfort and anxiety.

Disturbed sleep may be due to an increase in day-time sleep, inactivity, anxiety, depression, pain, physical discomfort, alcohol, tea and coffee. Some drugs, such as opioids (benzodiazepam), may cause nightmares, disrupted sleep or confusion. Steroids can cause general arousal and they should therefore be given in the morning and midday and definitely before 6 pm.

Where possible, try to remove any likely cause. Avoid drinking coffee and too much alcohol before going to sleep. Avoid day-time sleeps if necessary.

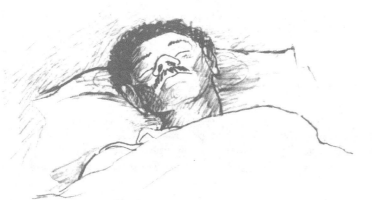

The following sedative agents are recommended:

◆ Benzodiazepines, such as oxazepam (Serepax), lorazepam (Ativan) or diazepam (Valium).

◆ Haloperidol (Serenace) can be used in more severe cases of anxiety and is very useful for controlling hallucinations.

Other useful sedatives include:

◆ Temazepan (Euhypnos, Normison), triazolam (Halcion) and midazolam (Dormicum).

Managing a patient who is dying

Caring for someone who is dying can be a difficult and trying time for a health care worker. It can also be rewarding and fulfilling. It is beyond the scope of this book to outline the process in detail.

The following is a brief outline of some of the more important considerations:

◆ Health care workers need to feel confident

It is important for the health care workers themselves to be comfortable with caring for people in the process of dying. They must be prepared to face the challenge. If the health care worker is scared or afraid of death or uncomfortable talking about death, then these fears and uncertainties will be conveyed to the patient and the family.

You, as the health care worker, will need to become familiar with managing dying people and be able to approach the issue with confidence. This may mean exploring your own feelings, fears, worries and inadequacies. You may need to set up a discussion or support group with other health care workers to discuss these issues, to clarify your own feelings and to develop counselling skills *(see Chapter 13).*

> **If the health care worker is scared or afraid of death or uncomfortable talking about death, then these feelings will be conveyed to the patient and the family.**

◆ Patient and family involvement

Include the patient and the family in the process and avoid denying the 'truth' of the situation.

Try to involve the patient, the close relatives and friends in the process. This usually means being open and honest and including the patient and the relatives in decisions and plans. This often needs adequate time and patience.

Be open to talking to the patient and close relatives about fears, worries, concerns and dying.

It is not good to avoid discussing or denying the fact that the patient is dying. This will create an environment of 'silence' which is unhelpful and usually creates more fear and anxiety. People are often more afraid of the unknown than the known.

Patients and their family often want to, and need to, talk about dying. This serves to express feelings and fears and helps to prevent anxiety and other problems. Being open about death can help the patient and his/her loved ones get close and make the dying process a very meaningful and enriching process. It also helps to prevent 'regrets' that later make the grieving process more difficult for the relatives.

Leading questions

It may be necessary to ask a few leading questions to give the patient, or the family members, an opportunity to express their feelings, e.g.

◆ **Health care worker:**

"You seem to be anxious and worried? ...
would you like to tell me what is on your mind?"

"Would you like to share some of your thoughts?"

"What do you think is going to happen to you?"

"You seem to be afraid of something ...
would you like to tell me about it?"

"Your mind seems to be disturbed today
... is there something worrying you?"

"Do you have any fears?"

Questions like these need to be dealt with sensitively and carefully. Sometimes you may need to choose the right time to ask these questions.

◆ **Often the patient or family will give clues about dying, e.g.**

Patient:

"Do you think I will ever improve or get better?"

◆ **Symbolic language may be used, e.g.**

Patient:

"Last night I went on a long journey."

"My train is waiting for me."

"I am going home soon."

Take care not to read this kind of language as nonsense. It is often referring to dying and transcending to another place. Rather explore it with the patient, e.g.

Health care worker:

"What is important for you about going home?"

"Where is the train going to take you?"

♦ **Sometimes the patient or family will express their concerns in other ways.**
They may become withdrawn or depressed, have sleep problems, nightmares, loss of appetite.

Patients may also deny the reality by avoiding the subject or talking about their long-term future plans or "when I am better" etc. This can be difficult to manage as it may be one of the ways the patient copes with the problem. However, it will deny him/her the opportunity to share worries and fears etc. Also they may say such things to test you (the health care worker). Sometimes they hope you will go along with it and give hope of an improvement or long-term survival.

♦ **It is important to explore with the patient what he/she is saying in more detail, e.g.**

Patient:

"When I get better will I ...?"

Health care worker:

"Are you asking if I think you will get better?"

or

"Are you saying you believe you are going to get better?"

or

"Do you feel you are getting better?"

or

"It seems you still have much you want to do or say. How can I help you?"

Sometimes you will need to decide whether to allow the patient to continue denying the reality of the situation. This may be best for some people. However, experts in this field stress the importance of usually facing the reality and dealing with it in a constructive manner.

Patients and their family often want to, and need to, talk about dying. Be open while talking to the patient and close relatives about fears, worries, concerns and dying. It is not good to avoid discussing, or denying, the fact that the patient is dying (to the patient or the family). This creates an environment of 'silence' which is unhelpful and in turn creates more fear and anxiety.

◆ The health care workers must be readily available

It is important for the patient and family to know that you, the health care worker, will be available and easily and readily approachable for any problems or concerns. The dying patient must never fear being left alone or abandoned by the health carer or the family. The patient must know where or how to get hold of you in times of need. Part of the therapeutic process is 'popping in' to see the family and patient regularly and making it clear that you care and will be available if needed.

Health care workers often feel that they have nothing more to offer if there is no possibility of curative therapy or if the medical situation is irreversible. However, often just being with the patient, and listening to concerns and worries and showing empathy etc. is itself very meaningful and therapeutic for the patient and family.

> **A patient must know that he / she will not be left alone or abandoned by close relatives and by the health care worker.**

◆ Treat pain, discomfort, sleep problems, anxiety etc.

Pain, discomfort, anxiety and sleep disorders can usually be effectively treated (*see pages 293 – 303*). It is unnecessary and bad for the family and patient if these problems are not effectively managed. There is no need for a patient to lie in pain or to have long, sleepless, anxiety-ridden nights.

- ◆ The use of opiates, such as morphine in a tablet or suspension, or even as a constant subcutaneous infusion may help to stop terror and pain.

- ◆ An intravenous infusion will also help, but this is rarely used.

- ◆ Benzodiazepines (such as diazepam) or propranolol will also decrease anxiety and fear.

- ◆ You may also need to advise and assist the family with some of the patient's problems, such as bedwetting / soiling, eating etc. A urinary catheter may be needed to avoid continual bed wetting. Plastic sheeting, undercovers or nappies (diapers) may also be needed for faecal soiling. Bed pans or urine bottles may also need to be made available.

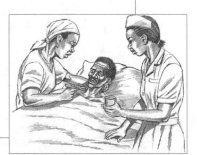

◆ Is the environment suitable?

The environment in which the patient is dying is very important. Where possible ensure that the patient is comfortable, clean, dignified, warm and safe.

Is the environment suitable? Would the patient prefer being at home or in a hospital?

Is the patient lonely or being left alone? Are the family providing appropriate support and can this be further encouraged and improved?

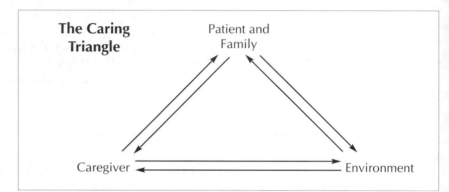

The Caring Triangle

Patient and Family

Caregiver

Environment

◆ Counselling for the family

Family, friends and lovers may also need counselling and care.

It is easy to forget about the needs of others close by. Often a husband, wife, lover, child or close friend is suffering from anxiety, fear, depression and stress. Keep a look-out for signs of these problems and try to provide care, support and counselling.

Involvement of other agencies and health care workers

◆ A team approach

If possible involve other terminal care agencies, such as hospice associations, cancer associations and AIDS organisations, to assist in managing a dying patient. Social workers, clinical psychologists, bereavement counsellors etc. are often experienced in dealing with these issues and can be very helpful.

A team approach in caring for a dying person and his/her family is best. Usually one person should take the responsibility/leadership and ensure that there is adequate co-ordination of the team. The primary care doctor or nurse is often in the best position to assume this role.

◆ Spiritual care

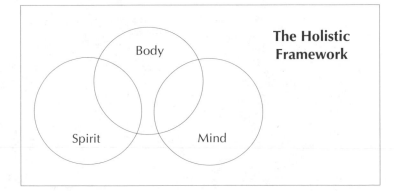

The body and mind are not the only areas which need care. Often there is a need for spiritual support as well. Include and encourage the involvement of any relevant or appropriate religious organisation or minister in the above team. Avoid suggesting this to the patient as it frequently creates anxiety related to imminent death. The requests should initially come from the patient.

The Holistic Framework

Body

Spirit

Mind

◆ Traditional healers

Traditional healers can play an important role and should be encouraged if appropriate.

◆ Health worker – heal thyself

Managing people who are dying can be very stressful for the health workers. Health workers should try to arrange for regular support and discussion groups to express anxieties and difficulties and share these with colleagues.

Occasionally the health worker may need to seek supportive counselling and supervision from experienced colleagues or counsellors.

"Time out" and having occasional breaks away from patient care is important to help maintain good mental health and enthusiasm.

> **Many dying patients will be adequately comforted and 'sedated' with the knowledge that friends and family are nearby. They need to know that they will not be abandoned or left alone, that their medical needs are understood and that the health care worker is confident and competent to deal with any 'emergency' calmly and skilfully.**
>
> **A caring and concerned health care worker who will listen to the patient will create an atmosphere which will promote acceptance of dying and death. Keeping the patient clean and dignified, in an acceptable environment, and free from pain and anxiety will help to allow the process to be calm and meaningful to the patient and the family.**

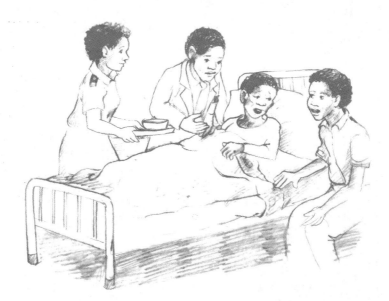

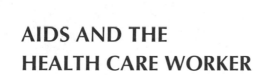

Chapter 15

AIDS AND THE HEALTH CARE WORKER

The role of the health care worker

HIV infection and health care workers

Accidental injury to the health care worker

Precautions to avoid contracting HIV infection
from patients

Precautions to prevent the spread of HIV infection to other
patients or health care workers

The role of the health care worker

AIDS has created new challenges and new problems for health care workers

- Health care workers are expected to provide the care for HIV-infected people.

- They are expected also to be role models regarding the proper acceptance of HIV-infected people with the necessary respect and dignity.

- They are also expected to teach people about the epidemic and its prevention.

For caregivers, AIDS has raised many ethical and moral issues, especially relating to the proper conduct and fair treatment of people with HIV/AIDS. AIDS is also a serious life-threatening and usually terminal condition. Health care workers are being asked to provide both physical and emotional support and care for those dying.

The very small risk of acquiring the HIV infection from a sharp instrument injury, such as a needle or scalpel blade, has created a new risk to caregivers. Precautions are needed to avoid this risk.

As teachers, health care workers have to understand clearly how HIV is, and is not, spread. HIV is not spread from casual contact, such as coughing, breathing, touching, laughing, towels, toilets, baths, eating utensils, clothes, etc. If health workers do not accept these facts, then we cannot expect acceptance from the general public.

Some of the ethical and moral issues are discussed below.

◆ The ethical and moral conduct of health workers who care for people with HIV/AIDS

There have been many misconceptions, myths, untruths and bad information about AIDS. Fear and hysteria have been spread about the disease.

People with HIV/AIDS have been unfairly blamed, discriminated against, rejected and alienated.

Health workers have also been influenced by much of this negative and damaging information. Many have allowed their own prejudices or moral values to influence their care of people with HIV/AIDS. Often this has resulted in the unfair and bad treatment of people infected with HIV.

Needle and other sharp instrument injuries with HIV-infected blood may be a **small** risk to health care workers, but this is the only real risk. There is no need to fear treating people with HIV/AIDS as it is possible to avoid accidental infection if some simple precautions are taken *(these are discussed on pages 328 – 333).*

People with HIV infection must be received and treated with respect, dignity and sensitivity.

◆ Some important ethical and moral guidelines when caring for people with HIV/AIDS

◆ **Receive all patients with the same respect, dignity, sensitivity and kindness** as you would for any other patient. HIV/AIDS can be very distressing and disturbing for someone to cope with. It is particularly important that health care workers make the lives of these patients easier. They must not add to their burden by making their lives more difficult.

A patient with HIV infection was heard to say, "I can usually cope with being HIV-infected and becoming ill, but I cannot cope with the bad attitude of people towards me."

◆ **It is important not to judge the moral values of your patients.** Take care not to lay blame or discriminate against people with HIV/AIDS. Avoid any form of rejection or alienation of such patients. Do not allow some of your own moral values and prejudices to influence your care of patients (your values may differ from those of the patient).

◆ New therapies can now offer people with HIV more hope and a better outlook. Health care workers must be familiar with new developments, and they must offer their patients the opportunity to consider these new therapies.

◆ **Strict and absolute confidentiality is always required.** Avoid discussing the details of the patient with anyone else, unless the information is necessary for the adequate care of the patient. It is acceptable to inform another health care worker whether a patient is HIV positive only if this worker is directly caring for, or about to care for, the patient. A person's HIV status is not for public information or for the indiscriminate use of any other health care worker.

◆ **It is unacceptable and unethical to refuse to treat a person just because they are HIV infected**. It is unethical to withhold certain accepted treatment procedures or practices. The best possible care must be provided.

◆ **Patients with HIV/AIDS have the right to privacy.** The health care worker must respect this privacy at all times.

◆ **Special considerations are required when you do HIV tests on patients**. Having an HIV test may dramatically change the life of a person. A positive result can create many social and psychological problems and a negative result may lead a person to believe that he / she is 'immune' or 'safe' from acquiring HIV infection.

People have the right to an **informed choice** as to whether or not to undergo the test. This means that they have the **right to refuse to have a test**. Health workers need to provide information and explanations about the test and provide the necessary counselling before and after the test *(see Chapters 4 and 13)*.

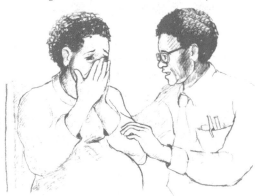

◆ **Health care workers who are HIV positive themselves should not do invasive surgical procedures on others.** It is recommended that an HIV-positive health care worker should consult a colleague, who is experienced with HIV/AIDS, to help make the decision as to whether it is acceptable or not to carry out certain medical procedures.

The rest of this chapter deals with the risk for health care workers of acquiring HIV infection and what to do if injured by an instrument which is contaminated with HIV-positive blood. The various precautions to avoid getting HIV infection or spreading it in the health care workplace will be outlined on the following page.

HIV infection and health care workers

◆ How a health care worker may become HIV infected in the workplace

HIV can be transmitted to a health care worker if:

◆ The worker is injured with a sharp instrument (such as needles, blades, broken glass) **and** if the instrument is contaminated with HIV-positive blood. The injury must penetrate the skin.

◆ HIV-positive blood enters the body of the health care worker through an open fresh wound or fresh sores on the skin or mucous membranes.

Remember the HIV-positive blood needs to enter directly into the body.

Most injuries with sharp instruments do not effectively transmit the HIV virus.

It is very **uncommon** for the HIV virus to be transmitted through needle and other sharp instrument injuries. It has been shown that there is only approximately a 1 in 330 chance of getting HIV infection from such an injury.

In almost all reported cases of HIV transmission from needle injuries, the injury was deep and penetrating and from a hollow-bore needle. This usually means that there is a very small chance that a worker will be infected from usual injuries, but it is best to avoid even this small chance.

Very few doctors, nurses or laboratory workers have become infected through their work. The newspapers tend to make big news out of these few cases and it may seem that lots of health care workers are being infected, but this is not true.

Most needle and other sharp instrument injuries with HIV-contaminated blood do not effectively transmit the virus to health care workers. But you need to take care to avoid even this small risk.

Accidental injury to the health care worker

◆ Guidelines for health care workers

The following guidelines are for health care workers who injure themselves with needles and other sharp instruments which may contain HIV-infected blood and other body fluids.

Risk of HIV transmission from accidental injury

Background information

Health care workers are at risk of accidental injury and exposure to HIV-infected blood and body fluids. There is an increased risk for those whose work is involved with taking blood, putting up drips or using sharp instruments such as needles, scalpels, insertion of intravenous drips, minor and major surgery, obstetrics, dental work etc. Laboratory workers are also at risk when handling blood products. Other potential infections can also be transmitted such as syphilis, malaria, hepatitis B etc.

It is important to know that the risk of getting HIV infection from a needle injury is generally very low. The average risk of HIV infection from all types of reported injuries through the skin (percutaneous) is 0,3%. This means approximately 1 in every 330 injuries will result in an established HIV infection in the health care worker.

The risk of infection has been found to increase if:

◆ The injury is deep i.e. it clearly penetrates the skin.

◆ There is visible blood on the needle or the instrument causing the injury.

◆ The needle / device was previously placed in the source patient's vein or artery i.e. the patient on whom the procedure was being carried out.

◆ The source patient had advanced HIV disease (AIDS). This means the source patient has:

    – a high viral load (*see page 74*)

    – or signs of HIV disease (*see pages 102 – 103*)

    – or a low CD4 cell count (*see page 73*)

The risk discussed on the previous page is considered to be higher than 0,3% if:

- a large volume of blood innoculated the health care worker;

- the source patient has a very high HIV viral load.

Note: Skin injuries via syringe needles (hollow-bore needles) seem to be the most common and risky sharp instruments for causing HIV infection through workplace injuries. Solid needles (not hollow-bored), such as a suturing needle, carry a lower risk.

> **The risk of an HIV infection from a needle injury is approximately 1 for every 330 injuries.**

Risk of HIV transmission from mucous membrane or skin exposure

The risk after mucous membrane (via the mouth) or skin exposure (without any injury) depends on the volume of blood and load of HIV in the blood (HIV viral load). However this risk is much lower and is reported to be approximately 0,1% and less than 0,1% respectively.

The risk from skin exposure (e.g. a skin splash, not an injury) is likely to be higher if:

- there is contact with the skin for a long time;

- the contact involves a large area of skin;

- the skin is unhealthy i.e. open wounds, diseased, inflamed, etc.;

- there is a high HIV viral load in the source patient's blood.

Note: A high HIV titre (viral load) in the source patient's blood is usually associated with the following:

- advanced immune-deficiency (low CD4 cell count)
- the AIDS phase of the HIV disease
- very early HIV infection (i.e. within the first few weeks after the initial infection)

The HIV viral titre may also rise during infections such as active tuberculosis (*see also diagram on page 76*).

◆ Role of anti-retrovirals (ARVs) in preventing HIV infection

In recent years there has been evidence that ARVs (such as AZT, 3TC, protease inhibitors) can significantly reduce the risk of HIV infection (sero-conversion) from percutaneous exposure to HIV-infected blood.

Post-exposure prophylaxis (PEP) can reduce the risk of HIV infection

It is recommended to give HIV-exposed health care workers ARVs to help prevent the HIV infection. This form of prophylaxis has become known as post-exposure prophylaxis (PEP).

PEP with zidovudine (AZT) alone was associated with a 79% reduction in risk of HIV infection after percutaneous exposure to HIV-positive blood. Some failures with PEP have occurred.

For HIV to successfully enter and establish itself in the body (from percutaneous or sexual transmission), it needs to be taken up by, and presented to, certain immune cells in the body. This process takes from several hours to several days. This provides an opportunity for ARV prophylaxis. The sooner this prophylaxis is started, the better the chance of reducing viral replication, and preventing the virus from establishing an ongoing infection in the body.

> **Post-exposure prophylaxis is best given as soon as possible after the injury – within the first hour or two.**

Every effort should be made to minimise the likelihood of viral replication occurring in the exposed health care worker. The following is required:

- rapid assessment of the exposure;
- PEP therapy with ARV drugs (e.g. ACT, 3TC) must start as soon as possible after the incident, and preferably within a few hours.

Post-exposure prophylaxis is not always successful

PEP failure may be due to the following:

◆ It may be due to exposure from HIV viral strains which are resistant to the drug regimen. Such resistant strains are more likely in patients who have previously been on ART.

◆ There may be a high HIV viral load in the source patient.

◆ The PEP may have been given too late or for insufficient duration.

Choice of ARV agents for PEP

◆ In HIV-infected patients combination therapy with nucleosides, such as zidovudine (AZT) and lamivudine (3TC), has greater ARV activity than zidovudine alone.

◆ This combination therapy is active against many zidovudine-resistant HIV strains without significantly increased toxicity.

◆ Adding a protease inhibitor (e.g. indinavir, saquinovir, ritonavir) provides even greater increase in ARV activity.

◆ Nevirapine should not be used for PEP.

Toxicity and possible side effects of ARVs used for PEP

◆ In currently recommended doses **zidovudine** is usually well tolerated by health care workers:

  – short-term toxicity associated with higher doses primarily includes gastro-intestinal symptoms (nausea, vomiting, diarrhoea, abdominal discomfort), fatigue and headache;

  – prolonged use (more than 1 – 3 months) may be associated with bone marrow suppression, however PEP is recommended for 4 weeks.

◆ **3TC** is known to cause gastro-intenstinal symptoms and rarely pancreatitis.

◆ **Protease inhibitor** side effects include hyperbilirubinaemia, kidney`stones and hyperglycaemia *(see also pages 88 – 92).*

◆ Other ARV drugs may also be recommended in the future as more information becomes available.

◆ Managing needle injury exposure to HIV-infected blood / fluids

The following recommendations will need to be reviewed on a regular basis and updated and adapted with any new relevant research or clinical experience.

Exposures that require the recommended management:

◆ A blood-contaminated needlestick injury

◆ Injury with another sharp instrument contaminated with blood, semen, CSF, pleural or other serous fluid (excluding urine and faeces)

◆ An occupationally-acquired, large exposure of the above fluids to the mucous membranes (eye, mouth)

◆ An occupationally-acquired blood splash onto broken or diseased skin (such as a 'weeping' excema)

The following management is recommended:

Clean the area immediately

◆ Clean the area immediately with an antiseptic solution.

◆ Rinse out the eye or mouth if these areas are exposed.

◆ Allow any wound to bleed freely for a few minutes.

Try to determine the HIV status of the source patient's blood

An attempt should be made, as soon as possible, to determine the HIV status of the source patient. If there is no record of the HIV status of the source patient, then an attempt should be made to obtain blood from the patient for this purpose.

This should be done in a proper and ethical manner with pre- and post-test counselling given to the patient.

In an urgent situation a reliable rapid HIV test could be done for this. This should be confirmed by a formal laboratory test thereafter.

The source patient should be given the option of receiving or not receiving the result of the test.

If the patient refuses to have his / her blood taken for an HIV test, and if there is no record of a recent HIV test result, then a doctor caring for the patient should be consulted as to the likelihood of the patient being HIV positive.

Alternatively there may be some of the patient's blood in the laboratory, if other blood tests were done:

      – this blood can be tested for HIV (only for the purposes of deciding on the need for PEP);

      – this information must then only be kept by the health care worker.

Clinical signs indicating a higher likelihood of HIV infection include:

◆ TB infection

◆ Signs of immune-deficiency such as oral thrush (candidiasis) and / or hairy leukoplakia on the tongue, recent herpes zoster or molluscum contagiosum infection, Kaposi's sarcoma etc.

◆ History of recurrent infectious conditions such as diarrhoeal diseases, pneumonia, meningitis, skin sepsis

◆ Unexplained weight loss

◆ Seborrhoeic dermatitis

◆ Persistent glandular lymphadenopathy

The above signs may help determine whether the source patient is likely to have HIV (in the absence of a blood test).

An HIV-positive source patient

◆ If the source patient is HIV positive, then start post-exposure prohylaxis (PEP) with ARV drugs immediately.

◆ ARV PEP is recommended if:

  – the source patient is HIV positive
  – the rapid HIV test is positive
  – in the absence of this information, if the source patient has one or more of the clinical signs suggesting HIV infection (*see previous page*).

◆ If the source patient's HIV status is unknown, consider PEP if:

  – the patient has one or more signs of HIV infection (*see previous page*)
  and / or
  – there is a blood-contaminated needlestick injury in an area with a high HIV prevalence amongst the community (*see page 324*).

Recommendations for post-exposure prophylaxis (PEP)

High risk exposures

PEP is recommended for any high risk exposures (*see page 323*). These include:

◆ Percutaneous injuries with sharp instruments contaminated with HIV-infected blood

◆ A large volume of blood contamination

◆ A deep injury

◆ A hollow-bore instrument injury (e.g. syringe needle previously in the source patient's vein or artery)

◆ Injected blood

◆ If the source patient has:

  – clinical AIDS
  – a high HIV RNA viral load
  – a low CD4 cell count

◆ PEP is also recommended for isolated risky sexual exposures such as post rape (*see page 219*).

HIV post-exposure prophylaxis regimens

◆ Basic 2-drug regimen

  – AZT 300 mg 12 hourly **plus** 3TC 150 mg 12 hourly for 28 days

◆ Alternative regimen

  – 3TC 150 mg 12 hourly **plus** d4T 40 mg 12 hourly

Expanded regimen (if severe contamination or potential drug resistance in source patient)

◆ one of the regimens from the previous page **plus**
  - Indinavir 800 mg 8 hourly
  - Nelfinavir 750 mg 8 hourly or 1250 mg 12 hourly
  - Efavirenz 600 mg daily
  - Abacavir 300 mg 12 hourly

Note: Neveripine should not be used for PEP as fatal liver failure has been reported.

The following table is a guide as to the 'strength' of the exposure and the recommendation:

PERCUTANEOUS INJURY	RISK OF EXPOSURE	RECOMMENDATION FOR PEP
Superficial injury	Increased	Consider ART
Visible blood on the needle	High risk	Strongly recommend ART
Needle used in a vein or artery	High risk	Strongly recommend ART
Deep intramuscular injury or injection into the body	Highest risk	Highly recommend ART
Source patient has clinical AIDS and / or a low CD4 cell count and / or a high viral load	Highest risk	Highly recommend ART
MUCOSAL AND SKIN CONTACTS	RISK OF EXPOSURE	RECOMMENDATION FOR PEP
Unbroken healthy skin	Low risk	Not recommended
Small volume and brief contact	Low risk	Consider ART
Large volume and / or prolonged contact	Increased	Recommend ART

Initiation of PEP

◆ PEP should be initiated promptly, preferably immediately, but within 1 – 2 hours after the exposure.

◆ The interval after which there is no benefit from using PEP is not yet defined.

◆ Some experts still consider PEP 7 – 14 days after the exposure in cases where there are highest risk exposures.

Duration of PEP

◆ PEP should be continued for 4 weeks provided there are no serious drug toxicities.

◆ If this occurs PEP may need to be discontinued.

Low risk exposures

◆ PEP can be *offered* to the health care worker in low risk exposures, (i.e. non-penetrating exposures) such as blood or other body fluid exposures to normal healthy skin, eye and mouth contamination. However this is not a strong recommendation.

◆ For urine and faecal contamination PEP is not recommended.

Unknown patient status

If the source patient's HIV status is not known, each case must be carefully considered before initiating PEP. This must be based on the exposure risk and likelihood of HIV infection in known or possible source patients.

Documentation of the health worker's HIV status

◆ An HIV blood test should be done and documented on the exposed health care worker at baseline (i.e. within 24 hours of the injury), at 6 weeks, 12 weeks and at 6 months
  – in rarer instances seroconversion can take place over a longer period than 6 months

◆ Tests for hepatitis B and C, syphilis, malaria etc. could also be considered.

◆ PCR and P24 antigen tests are not generally recommended as false positive and negative tests can occur. They may be used in specific situations (e.g. window period).

Supportive counselling should be available to the health care worker if required.

The health care worker should also consider using a barrier method for safe sexual practice until the above HIV tests are completed.

Avoidance of pregnancy in female health care workers is also recommended until seroconversion is excluded.

Condoms should be provided for this period, if necessary.

Monitoring of the health care worker

If PEP is initiated, the health care worker should be seen and monitored by a clinician who has experience in HIV care.

Side effects / toxicity of some of the drugs used in PEP

Side effects in healthy individuals are not common. Initially there may be some discomfort (nausea, vomiting, diarrhoea, headache) on commencing therapy, but this usually disappears after a few days.

◆ AZT side effects
  – headache, gastro-intestinal symptoms (nausea, vomiting, diarrhoea, indigestion)
  – more serious side effects, such as marrow suppression with resultant anaemia or pancytopaenia, are extremely rare in a healthy individual on short-course therapy (4 weeks). These usually only occur after prolonged use (more than 3 months).

◆ 3TC side effects
  – gastro-enteritis and rarely pancreatitis (epigastric pain, nausea and a raised serum amylase) usually happens after long-term use

- ◆ Indinavir side effects
  - – gastro-intestinal symptoms
  - – rarely renal stones (it is important to drink lots of fluids while on this drug)

If there is sero-conversion of the HIV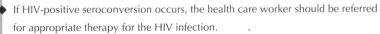

- ◆ If HIV-positive seroconversion occurs, the health care worker should be referred for appropriate therapy for the HIV infection.

Report the injury

- ◆ An appropriate and confidential reporting system is needed to document the exposure and the details of the source patient and the health care worker.
- ◆ This is necessary for medico-legal purposes and for possible compensation and insurance claims.
- ◆ A COIDA claim (Compensation for Occupational Injuries and Diseases Act) may also be necessary if the worker seroconverts
  - – this must be done within 11 months of the injury.

Starter packs must be available

- ◆ Health care services must have ARV 'starter packs' immediately available at the clinics and hospitals. This is a 2 – 3 day supply of the PEP drugs.
- ◆ 'Starter packs' of PEP drugs should be available in all health care services for the immediate initiation of PEP if necessary.

Policy and procedure

- ◆ Health care services should delegate responsible managers to ensure the correct reporting and recording procedures for occupational acquired HIV exposure.
- ◆ All health care workers including the cleaners, laboratory staff and anyone else who may come into contact with blood and body fluids should be aware of the process and procedure.

An HIV-negative source patient

- ◆ If the HIV test on the source patient is negative, then it can be assumed that there is an insignificant risk of exposure to HIV. This can only be assumed if there is reasonable information to suggest that the source patient is **not** in the window period.
- ◆ No further action is required in this case except to report the incident.

See Flow Chart on the following page.

> **As research into PEP progresses, other preferred ARV regimens may be recommended. Readers should keep up with the latest developments.**

THE HEALTH CARE WORKER

Prevention of HIV infection from occupationally acquired exposure to HIV

(For more details of routes of exposure, see 1 on opposite page)

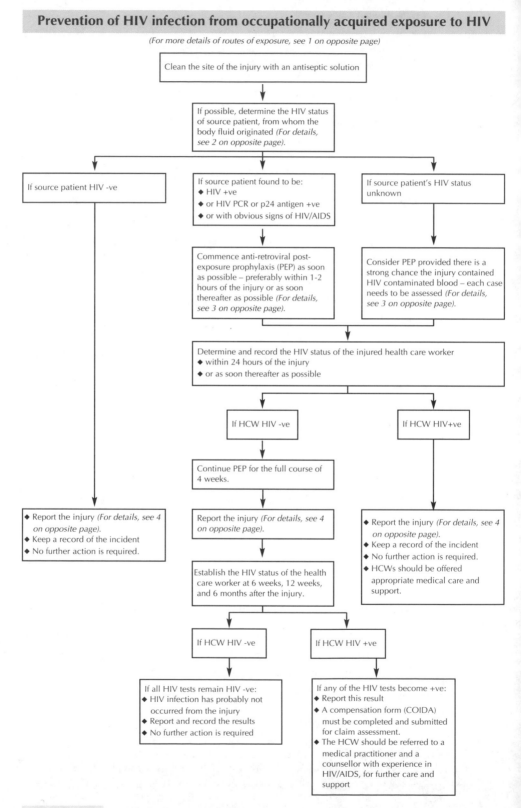

Clean the site of the injury with an antiseptic solution

↓

If possible, determine the HIV status of source patient, from whom the body fluid originated *(For details, see 2 on opposite page).*

If source patient HIV -ve

If source patient found to be:
♦ HIV +ve
♦ or HIV PCR or p24 antigen +ve
♦ or with obvious signs of HIV/AIDS

↓

Commence anti-retroviral post-exposure prophylaxis (PEP) as soon as possible – preferably within 1-2 hours of the injury or as soon thereafter as possible *(For details, see 3 on opposite page).*

If source patient's HIV status unknown

↓

Consider PEP provided there is a strong chance the injury contained HIV contaminated blood – each case needs to be assessed *(For details, see 3 on opposite page).*

Determine and record the HIV status of the injured health care worker
♦ within 24 hours of the injury
♦ or as soon thereafter as possible

If HCW HIV -ve

If HCW HIV+ve

↓

Continue PEP for the full course of 4 weeks.

♦ Report the injury *(For details, see 4 on opposite page).*
♦ Keep a record of the incident
♦ No further action is required.

Report the injury *(For details, see 4 on opposite page).*

♦ Report the injury *(For details, see 4 on opposite page).*
♦ Keep a record of the incident
♦ No further action is required.
♦ HCWs should be offered appropriate medical care and support.

Establish the HIV status of the health care worker at 6 weeks, 12 weeks, and 6 months after the injury.

If HCW HIV -ve

If HCW HIV +ve

If all HIV tests remain HIV -ve:
♦ HIV infection has probably not occurred from the injury
♦ Report and record the results
♦ No further action is required

If any of the HIV tests become +ve:
♦ Report this result
♦ A compensation form (COIDA) must be completed and submitted for claim assessment.
♦ The HCW should be referred to a medical practitioner and a counsellor with experience in HIV/AIDS, for further care and support

1. Treatment is highly recommended if a health care worker is exposed via:

◆ A penetrating injury by a blood-contaminated needle-stick
◆ An instrument contaminated with semen, cerebro-spinal fluid (CSF), pleural fluid or other serous fluids (not including faeces and urine)
◆ A skin or mucous membrane contamination that involves
  – a very large volume for a prolonged period of time
  – a large wound or unhealthy, diseased area
  – significant contamination of the eye or mouth

2. Determine the HIV status of source patient by the following methods:

◆ from the clinical records
◆ from any laboratory report
◆ by doing a rapid HIV antibody blood test (confirm an HIV +ve result with a laboratory-based test later)
◆ by doing a laboratory-based HIV antibody test
◆ by doing an HIV PCR or HIV p24 antigen test (only in special circumstances)

Note:
Any HIV test on the source patient must be done with informed consent and with adequate pre- and post-test counselling.

3. The following PEP regimen is recommended:

◆ AZT (zidovudine) 200 mg 8 hourly for 4 weeks
◆ 3TC (lamivudine) 150 mg 12 hourly for 4 weeks *(see also page 322)*

A starter pack should be available in the clinical setting to help with the early use of the above drugs. Consider adding indinavir i.e. Crixivan 800 mg 8 hourly for 4 weeks if the source patient has been receiving ART with AZT and 3TC as part of their usual treatment.

Note:
◆ In the absence of the above drugs, other anti-retroviral agents could be used. However at the moment there is not enough scientific evidence to suggest alternative regimens should be used.
◆ The health care worker may need to be counselled and followed up by a medical practitioner experienced in HIV/AIDS care.
◆ The health care worker will need to consider safe sexual practices until future tests prove that HIV was not transmitted through the injury.

4. A detailed report should include the following information:

◆ The time, place, nature and type of injury
◆ The circumstances of the injury
◆ The clinical condition of the source patient, especially relating to their HIV status and HIV-related signs and symptoms
◆ Any steps that were taken to obtain the source patient's HIV status (if it is refused)
◆ The HIV status of the health care worker at the time of the injury
◆ Any therapeutic action and details of medication that were taken
◆ Names of medical practitioners
◆ Record of any witnesses to the injury
◆ Record of the HIV status of the health care worker and the source patient

THE HEALTH CARE WORKER

Precautions to avoid contracting HIV infection from patients

People with HIV/AIDS should be cared for in the normal way. In most situations there is no need to isolate patients with HIV. In some instances the patient may have a potentially infectious disease, such as salmonella, shigella dysentery, a multi drug-resistant tuberculosis, a cryptosporidia infection etc. In these cases barrier/isolation care may be necessary.

The following simple precautions are needed:

The handling of used needles

Re-sheathing needles

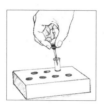

Injuries with syringe and drip needles (which are contaminated with HIV blood) are the most common cause of accidental HIV infection to health care workers.

The most common way in which needles injure workers is when the needle is being replaced into the protective cover (sheath).

It is important not to re-sheath or re-cover used needles unless there is a special apparatus which will hold the sheath and give the health worker protection.

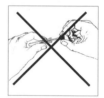

If a needle must be re-sheathed, then you must not hold the needle cover (sheath) with your other hand.
It is better to place the sheath in a sheath-holder, or on a flat surface, while you insert the needle into the sheath.

Discarding needles

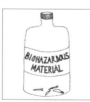

All needles must be discarded into protected containers.
Never discard a used needle or sharp instrument into a dustbin or paper or plastic bag.

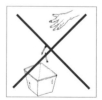

A sharp needle placed in an unprotected container may injure another person who is handling the container.

Do not re-sheath used needles.
Do not discard used needles or sharp instruments into dustbins or bags.

THE HEALTH CARE WORKER

Procedures that involve blood and body fluids

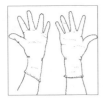

Wear gloves

Wear gloves when using sharp instruments, taking blood, putting up drips, handling contaminated materials, and for dressings and handling body fluids.

HIV cannot enter through normal intact (undamaged) skin but there is a small risk of it entering through very small cuts, sores or cracks in the skin. These small openings may not be seen. Take extra care to avoid blood splashing or spilling onto your skin. Also wash off any blood from your skin as soon as possible. **Keep obvious cuts and sores covered with waterproof plasters**.

Wear gloves when handling any blood-contaminated materials, such as swabs, cotton wool, bandages, dressings and instruments, or for handling any body fluids.

> **It is important to take precautions on ALL patients whether they are known to be HIV positive or not.**

Surgical procedures

The health care worker must take extra care when doing surgery, post-mortems and other invasive procedures.

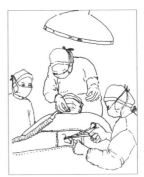

It is important to regard all patients as possibly being HIV infected, and to take precautions on them all. Take special care passing sharp instruments around during surgery. Also extra care should be taken when

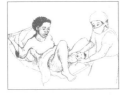

inserting or removing a blade from a scalpel. Workers doing post-mortem examinations should also take extra care.

Use gloves and a plastic apron if you are doing surgical procedures or delivering babies (childbirth).

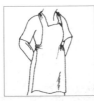
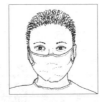
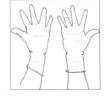

> **All protective items, such as gloves, masks, aprons etc., must be readily available in areas where these may be needed. Health workers have a right to safe working conditions.**

Washing hands

Always wash hands after examining or caring for a patient, after cleaning up, or after doing a procedure.

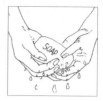

If possible use an antiseptic soap, such as iodine (Betadine), chlorhexidine (Hibitane / Hibiscrub) and cetrimide (Cetavlon, Savlon).

Other protective measures

Eye and mouth protection

Wear protective eye equipment (glasses or goggles) when doing procedures where body fluids may be splashed. This may occur during surgery, and for procedures such as lumbar punctures, incising abscesses, childbirth (rupturing membranes, delivery, cutting the umbilical cord, delivering the placenta, suturing tears and episiotomies etc.). This could also happen while emptying blood-containing drains and other containers.

HIV could possibly enter through the eye or mouth, expecially if there are sores or inflammation (although this has not yet been reported). It is best not to take any chances.

Health care workers should cover all cuts and abrasions with waterproof plasters.

Contaminated linen

Wear gloves and plastic aprons for handling contaminated linen, bedclothes, dressings, or for cleaning up any spills of blood or body fluids.

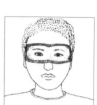

Mouth-to-mouth rescuscitation

There does not seem to be any serious risk of getting HIV infection through mouth-to-mouth resuscitation. If possible place a thin cloth over the mouth, to avoid any saliva or fluid exchange during mouth-to-mouth contact. However, it is best if you can use a manual ventilator, like an ambu bag.

Remember other workers, such as cleaners, must also wear protective clothing when handling contaminated materials.

Precautions to prevent the spread of HIV infection to other patients or health care workers

Health care workers can also pass on the HIV virus to other patients if they use contaminated instruments on patients.

Use needles or syringes only once

Never ever use the same needle or syringe on more than one patient.

Also never use the same immunization needle on more than one child. Always use a new needle and syringe or a clean sterile needle and instrument on each patient.

The sterilization of instruments is discussed below.

Only use sterile equipment and instruments

Use only sterile equipment for all procedures, such as anaesthesia, suturing and ventilating (breathing equipment etc.)

How to sterilize equipment

You can sterilize or destroy the HIV virus on any equipment by using **one** of the following means:

- Autoclave the instrument or needle.
- Boil the instrument or needle in boiling water for more than 30 minutes.
- Stand the instrument in 2% glutaraldehyde for 30 minutes.
- Stand the instrument in hypochlorite (chlorine) (10 000 ppm) for 30 minutes.
- If you do not have any of the above you can make a solution with household bleach (chlorine):
  - mix ¼ cup of bleach (or 2 tablespoons) with 2 cups of water;
  - soak instruments for at least 30 minutes.

Note:

The above disinfecting agents may not adequately disinfect the instrument if organic matter, such as blood, pus, body tissue etc., is left on the instrument. This means that instruments must be thoroughly cleaned before they are placed in the disinfectant agent.

Needles should be sterilized with heat (autoclaving or boiling) as the above disinfectants may not enter into the bore of the needle.

THE HEALTH CARE WORKER

Disposal of contaminated articles

Dispose of and transport contaminated material or body tissues safely.

- Dispose of sharp instruments, such as needles and blades, into a safe firm container. Label this 'Bio-hazardous material'.

- Syringes without needles should be thrown away into plastic bags.

- Soiled and contaminated linen must be discarded into special containers.

- Body tissues should be transported in firm sealed containers and labelled 'Bio-hazardous material'.

- It is best to rinse and clean all contaminated instruments before sending them off to the central sterilizing unit (CSSD).

- Remember also not to leave any blood or other body fluids on the outside of containers.

Cleaning body fluid contamination on surfaces

Avoid leaving spilled blood and any other body fluids lying around.

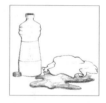

- Clean body fluid spills by covering the spill with a towel or cloth soaked in hypochlorite solution.

- For everyday cleaning of surfaces you can use hypochlorite/detergent 500 ppm (12 hypochlorite/detergent sachets in 5 litres of water).

- Simple household bleach (chlorine) can also be used to clean the spill and the surface. Use 1 cup of bleach mixed with 2 cups water. Pour onto the spill and mop up with a cloth or towel.

All blood for transfusion must be tested for HIV infection

Blood used for transfusion must be tested for HIV. Any blood showing antibodies should not be accepted for transfusion.

If blood is given in the 'window period' it may falsely test negative. This means that there is a very slight risk associated with blood transfusion. For this, and other reasons, **blood should only be given if it is life-saving or essential**.

Dealing with HIV-positive corpses

Remember to maintain all precautionary measures when handling dead bodies (corpses).

All health care workers **and** all other clinic or hospital personnel, such as cleaners, porters, clerks etc., must be educated and informed about AIDS. This should include the prevention of HIV in the workplace and spreading the disease to others.

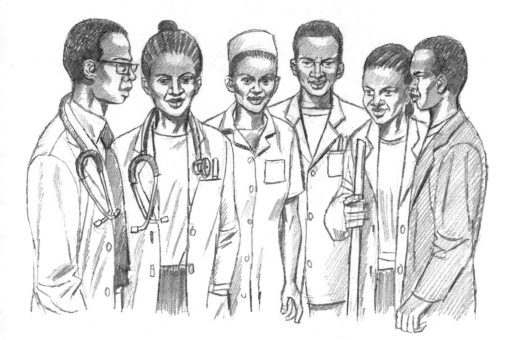

GLOSSARY

ABC	Abacavir
AIDS	Acquired immune-deficiency syndrome. This means the body has great difficulty in fighting infections because the immune system is weakened.
AIDS-defining disease	Specific diseases which, in the presence of HIV infection, indicate the clinical development of AIDS.
Antibodies	Special protein complexes produced by the immune system to fight against specific disease-causing organisms.
Anti-retroviral	Drugs which suppress or prevent replication of HIV
AROM	Artificial rupture of membranes during childbirth (labour)
ART	Anti-retroviral therapy
ARV	Anti-retroviral
AZT	Azidothymidine, also called zidovudine or Retrovir, an anti-retroviral drug
CD4 cells	These are T helper/inducer lymphocytes with CD4 receptors and are important cells which regulate and control aspects of the immune system. Also called T4 helper cells.
CD4 count	The laboratory test most commonly used to estimate the level of immune-deficiency (CD4 cells) in HIV infection.
CMV	Cytomegalovirus
COIDA	Compensation for Occupational Injuries and Diseases Act
d4T	Stavudine – an anti-retroviral drug
ddI	Didanosine
DOT	Directly observed therapy – a method used for treating tuberculosis patients
DTP	Diphtheria, tetanus, pertussis
EFV	Efavirenz
EIA	Enzyme-linked immunoassay
ELISA test	Enzyme-linked immunosorbant assay. A laboratory technique to detect antibodies in the blood.
Epidemiology	The study of the determinants, distribution, prevalence and control of diseases.
ESR	Erythrocyte sedimentation rate
False positive	A test result that is positive when the person is actually or truly negative.
False negative	A test result that is negative when the person is actually or truly positive.
FBC	Full blood count
FNA	Fine needle aspiration
FTA-ABS	Treponemal test (for syphilis)
HBV	Hepatitis B
HAART	Highly Active Anti-retroviral therapy
HiB	Haemophilus influenza type B
HIV	Human immuno-deficiency virus which causes AIDS
HIV antibody positive	Antibodies to HIV are present in the blood stream and this means that the person has been exposed to the HIV virus.
HIV positive	Refers to a person who has tested HIV positive and therefore has been exposed to the HIV virus and is infected with the virus.
HIV P24 antigen (**HIV antigen test**)	A core protein found in the HIV virus. The presence of this antigen is evidence of the HIV virus and is usually detectable in the early and very late stages of HIV infection.
HSV	Herpes simplex virus
IDV	Indinavir
Immune system	That part of the body's structure and function which fights against infections and other foreign recognised bodies.
Immune-deficiency	A weakening or deficiency in the immune system

Infection	Invasion and replication in the body of organisms, such as viruses, bacteria, fungi and parasites.
IUCD	Intra-uterine contraceptive device
KS	Kaposi's sarcoma – an unusual cancer of blood capillaries common in people with AIDS
LIP	Lymphoid interstitial pneumonia
LPV	Lopinavir
MAC/MAI	Mycobacteria avium / intracellulare complex
MDR	Multi drug-resistant tuberculosis
MMR	Mumps, measles, rubella
MTCT	Mother to child HIV transmission
NFV	Nelfinavir
NNRTI	Non-nucleoside reverse transcriptase inhibitor – a class of anti-retroviral drugs
NRTI	Nucleoside reverse transcriptase inhibitor – a class of anti-retroviral drugs
NVP	Nevirapine
Opportunistic infections	Infection of the body as a result of a weakening of the body's defence. These infections would not normally cause disease in a normal healthy body.
OHL	Oral hairy leukoplakia
OPV	Oral polio vaccine
PCP	*Pneumocystis carinii* pneumonia – an opportunistic infection causing pneumonia due to the Pneumocystis *carinii* organism.
PCR	Polymerase chain reaction – a method of testing for the presence of HIV in the body
PEP	Post-exposure prophylaxis
PI	Protease inhibitor – a class of anti-retroviral drugs
PID	Pelvic inflammatory disease
Retrovirus	A group of viruses, including HIV, which replicate by changing genetic RNA into the DNA of host's cells.
Reverse transcriptase	An enzyme which retroviruses produce and use in the replication process.
RPR	Rapid plasma reagin (syphilis test)
RTI	Reverse transcriptase inhibitor – a class of anti-retroviral drugs
RTV	Ritonavir
3TC/lamivudine	An anti-retroviral drug
Sero-conversion/ illness	The development of antibodies in response to infection. With HIV infection, it is associated with the development of an HIV positive antibody test, and there may be signs and symptoms of a non-specific illness (sero-conversion illness).
Shingles	Herpes zoster skin manifestation
SQV	Saquinavir
STI	Sexually transmitted infection
Syndrome	Range of different diseases, symptoms or conditions
T4 cell	See CD4 cells
TPHA	Treponemal test (for syphilis)
Unprotected sex	Sexual intercourse where there is a free potential for the exchange of the sexual fluids between partners.
VDRL	A non-specific syphilis test
Virus	A microbiological organism which is the smallest and most basic of the known organisms.
WB (Western blot test)	A highly accurate blood test for antibodies to HIV infection, usually used to confirm a positive HIV ELISA test.
'Window' period	The time between the initial (first) HIV infection and the development of detectable HIV antibodies. During this time the antibody test will be falsely negative. The test will be negative even though the person is actually infected with HIV.
ZDV	Zidovudine

INDEX